**IT'S NOT AS EASY AS I THOUGHT!**

# REVELATIONS ABOUT WORKING AND WELLNESS FROM A REAL WANDERER

Kristine Hudson

© 2020 It's Not As Easy As I Thought! Revelations About Working and Wellness from a Real Wanderer
All rights reserved. No part of the book may be reproduced in any shape or form without permission from the publisher.

This guide is written from a combination of experience and high-level research. Even though we have done our best to ensure this book is accurate and up to date, there are no guarantees to the accuracy or completeness of the contents herein.

This cover has been designed using resources from unsplash.com
ISBN: 978-1-953714-30-5

# Reviews

Reviews and feedback help improve this book and the author. If you enjoy this book, we would greatly appreciate it if you could take a few moments to share your opinion and post a review on Amazon.

## Also by Kristine Hudson

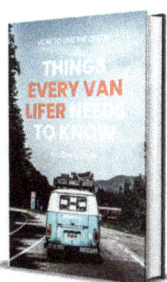

**Things Every Lifer Needs to Know**

mybook.to/vanlife

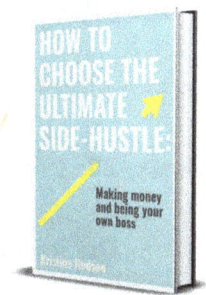

**How to Choose the Ultimate Side-hustle**

mybook.to/side-hustle

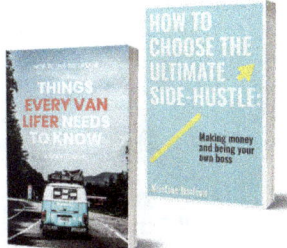

**The Modern Woman's Guide to Living Wild and Free**

mybook.to/vanbundle1

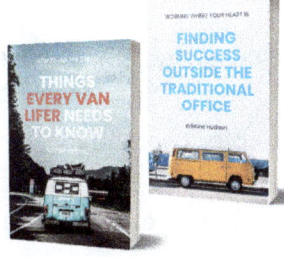

**Living and Prospering Wherever You Wish**

mybook.to/vanbundle2

# Work Where You Want to Be: How to Leave the Office Behind

## Section One: The Here and Now of Working on the Run — 11

   Introduction: Why Do I Need This Book? What Will I Learn? — 11

   Chapter One: My Own Journey to "Working on the Run" — 14

      Kristine's List — 22

   Chapter Three: The Pros & Cons of Working Remotely — 25

   Chapter Four: What Will You Accomplish With This Change? — 28

## Section Two: Details, Details, Details — 33

   Chapter One: Determining the Who, Where, When, and How of Working on the Run — 33

      Your Challenge: An Exercise in Reality — 34

   Chapter Two: Who, Where, and When- Just the Facts — 36

## Section Three: What Will I Be? What Will I Do? — 45

   Chapter One: Same as It Ever Was — 46

   Chapter Two: Redefining the "Free" in "Freelancing" — 52

   Chapter Three: A Side-Hustle You Can Do All Day- or Not! — 56

   Chapter Four: Here, There, and Everywhere — 61

   Chapter Five: Something for Everyone — 63

## Section Four: Setting the Stage   65

### Chapter One: Creating Your Work Space   65

### Chapter Two: Understanding How to Work in a New Place   70

### Chapter Three: Time to Work!   73

## Section Five: Finding Your Stride and Making It Work   79

### Chapter One: The Social Aspect   79

### Chapter Two: The Growth Aspect   83

### Chapter Three: The Financial Aspect   86

### Chapter Four: The Fear Aspect   88

## Section Six: Wrapping It All Up   95

### Section 6: Resources for Former Office Workers   101

- Productivity Management Resources   101

- Money Management Resources   102

- Technical Resources   103

- Network/Community Resources   106

# From Wheels to Wellness

**Section 1: Introduction** — 113

    Chapter 1: What You Need to Know — 115

    Chapter 2: What Do I Know? — 117

**Section 2: Taking Care of Your One and Only Body** — 121

    Chapter 1: Keeping Up with Preventive Care — 122

        A Few Words About Insurance — 127

    Chapter 2: Nutrition and Eating for You — 133

        The Importance of Proper Food Storage — 136

        Cooking for Your Crowd — 142

        A Drop About Hydration — 143

    Chapter 3: Exercise: "Moving More Than a Van" — 145

        Regular Activity for Those Who Wander — 148

        "Extended Driving Pose" Is Not An Exercise — 149

        Outside of the Outdoors — 151

**Section 3: Managing Less Than Perfect Health on the Road** — 157

    Disclaimer: This Book Is Not a Doctor — 158

    Chapter 1: Managing Chronic Conditions from Anywhere and Everywhere — 158

Be Open With Your Care Team ... 160

Medication Tips ... 161

Chapter 2: When Bad Things Happen ... 163

Preparing for Minor Disasters ... 163

What to Do When Things Get Worse ... 169

**Section 4: A Brief Section about Housekeeping and Hygiene ... 173**

Chapter 1: Basic Van Cleanliness ... 174

Chapter 2: Laundry Day! ... 176

Chapter 3: Clean Van, Clean You ... 177

**Section 5: Mental Health Matters ... 181**

Chapter 1: The Reality of Road Fatigue ... 182

But What If It's Worse Than That? ... 183

The Side Effects of Having Too Much Time to Think ... 186

Chapter 2: Finding and Continuing Mental Health Care on the Road ... 188

Chapter 3: When It Becomes Too Much ... 190

**Health and Wellness in 2020: Special Notes About COVID-19 Considerations ... 193**

**Conclusion ... 197**

**Resources ... 199**

WORKING WHERE YOUR HEART IS:

# WORK WHERE YOU WANT TO BE: HOW TO LEAVE THE OFFICE BEHIND

Kristine Hudson

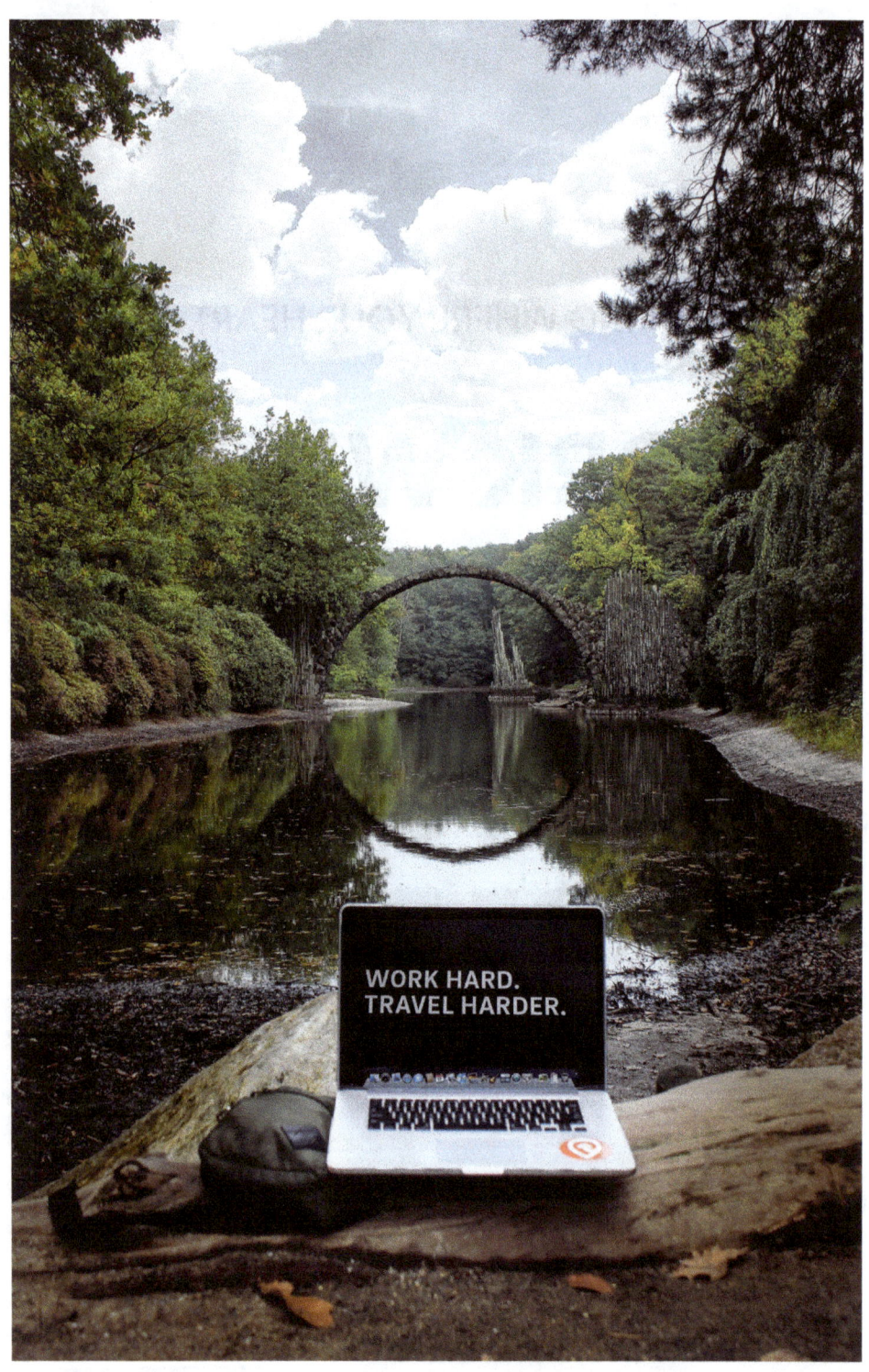

# Section One: The Here and Now of Working on the Run

## Introduction: Why Do I Need This Book? What Will I Learn?

Not too long ago, the concept of "working remotely" was reserved only for the lucky few. In fact, many larger corporations mistakenly believed that workers were most productive and provided the most value for the employers' investments when they were seated at a company-supplied desk, in a deliberately organized cubicle formation, with a corporate-issued phone and computer. Occasionally, a top-level executive would take his or her work on the road while attending a productivity conference half a world away. Perhaps, after a great deal of deliberation, an expecting mother would be given the access to log in while on bed rest. These situations were few and far between.

One may argue whether it was the general success of these work-from-home pioneers that paved the way for the modern trend of working remotely. Others point out that the catalyst of this movement was the resulting rebellion from those who asked "if they can do it, why can't we?" Though both parties have made valid contributions to the increasing number of people who telecommute to their jobs on a regular basis, much of the thanks can be attributed to ever-evolving technology and security protocols, which have made the notion of working from anywhere BUT a cubicle a more regular practice.

The phrase "working remotely" has evolved since the early days of being a rare privilege. While many think of it as "working from home," the truth is that technology has advanced light years in the past 30 years, which has taken the concept from just a home office, to almost anywhere as long as you can get a reliable phone signal (that can then be converted into a Wi-Fi Hotspot!).

The fact that we can work from anywhere offers endless possibilities. Not coincidentally, the number of individuals living the nomadic "van life" dream has also increased dramatically. For many people, the conclusion is obvious: the time has come to work on the road.

Now that you're considering working remotely, you're probably feeling refreshed and incredibly inspired by this imminent taste of freedom. You may feel ready to go. Just boot up your laptop, and the workday starts, right? Well, unfortunately it's not so simple.

In the following chapters, we are going to look at working remotely from the inside, out. Thanks to the early pioneers of the work from home, or "WFH" movement, today's workers can learn the intricacies, difficulties, rewards, and challenges of leaving the office behind. There are many reasons why one might choose to make this change and, whether you do so regularly or intermittently, it's a great idea to know what you're getting into before you take the leap.

Perhaps you are just starting to kick around the idea of working remotely. Maybe you're getting the sneaking suspicion that winding your way through endless traffic twice a day, only to stare at the same walls for the majority of your working hours isn't the way you want to live. Regardless of how much you love your job, a lot of your engagement level as an employee comes from the environment in which you work. If you find yourself overly stressed about your commute, your office space, your coworkers, or all of the above, your productivity will most likely decline. You may find yourself more focused on your emotional situation than the tasks you need to accomplish. At this stage, perhaps you're thinking about proposing the idea of working remotely to your manager, but you're not sure how to approach it, or if it would even be a good idea.

Or maybe that's not you at all. You may be perfectly happy working in the office. You could not be happier with your job, and you cherish the time you spend in your car, catching up on your favorite podcasts. Maybe the social aspect of your office inspires you. That being said, there may be something that frequently drags you away from the office. Maybe you have a child or family member who requires attention. It could be difficulties with your own health. You might just feel drawn to a lifestyle that involves a change of scenery. For any number of reasons, it's far more practical in your situation to step away from the office building and work where you are physically needed. You might be wondering if this is the right decision, and how you can get all your ducks in a row before you start moving things out of your cubicle.

Then again, you may have already jumped ahead to the "remote" part, and now you need to pick up on the "working" thing. It's not unusual to put the cart before the horse- or in this case, the van before the bank account. Some folks quit their jobs for a life of adventure, enjoy a span of freedom, then gradually return to the working world once their money situation becomes too tight.

There's no "one true way" to do WFH, just as there isn't a "correct" van lifestyle or one "perfect" way to do any given job. In fact, you may have absolutely no desire to live in a van or travel the roads — you just want to have the option available if that desire did arise. For some, the freedom of working remotely may be working at the very edge of the 5G service areas. Others may reflect that freedom by wearing a bathrobe and sipping iced tea on the back porch while conducting a meeting.

Your ideal setup might be working from a designated work space within your home. WFH is a great situation for many people. You might want to have the flexibility to work from anywhere, or "work remotely." Some larger companies offer an option they term "telecommuting," which gives you the advantage of never directly working with anyone- you simply call in whenever necessary and otherwise submit work via email or cloud. Many remote workers are even able to alternate between these different forms. One day might be spent at the home office, another might be spent on the road while heading to client onsite meetings, and other days might be spent tied to the telephone.

Regardless of where you want to work, the concepts of working on the run are shared amongst nearly everyone who is ready to walk away from the cube farm and into the world of earning an income from literally anywhere else. Whether you're setting up office from the back of your converted skoolie, or from your Manhattan apartment, many of the following tips will be helpful for transitioning successfully. In this book, we'll cover many common concerns, including connectivity and scheduling. We'll take a look at how to set up a workspace that helps you stay productive and inspired as well as maintaining peace of mind and reducing stress throughout the transition. You may not have considered how your life will change once you introduce work into your living situation, but you will likely experience some significant physical, mental, and psychological shifts.

Though transitioning from a static office job to work on the run is very, very rewarding for many people, it's also a decision not to be taken lightly. There are preparations to be made throughout every aspect of your life. This is especially true if you are coordinating your work transition with other life changes. While some of these may be intuitive to a seasoned office worker, many of us are not aware of what we take for granted until something goes awry. The purpose of this book is to keep you focused and mindful of those things which can be complicated, challenging, or not yet apparent.

Working on the run is not for everyone. By reading this book, you will be able to better determine whether your work style and lifestyle are conducive to working outside of the office environment, office hours, or both. After we've discussed the considerations of making the transition, we'll go over the job options best suited to a nomadic lifestyle, and strategies on conditioning your mind and environment to help you become your most productive self, no matter how distracting your surroundings may be. Working remotely requires a lot of self-discipline, but for those with the right attitude and preparation, it can be one of the best decisions of your life.

**Chapter One: My Own Journey to "Working on the Run"**
In retrospect, there's nothing in my upbringing that would've suggested that I would choose the type of lifestyle I've chosen. Starting from a young age, my parents made it a point to take me on exciting adventures several times a year.

Sometimes we'd journey via plane from our home in Ohio to highly exotic locations (at least, in my young and impressionable eyes), such as the seashores of Florida. We once stayed at a friend's condo, where I was completely entertained by the tiny lizards that would zip around the patios and sidewalks. This may seem super mundane for many readers, but for a preschooler from the suburbs, this was an amazing experience.

Other journeys were less exotic but still offered excitement with the added bonus of being educational. We'd visit museums in Columbus, Cleveland, and Cincinnati. We would drive down to the American South to visit family members for the holidays and watch the brisk Northern weather warm through car windows that would eventually be rolled down as the temperatures climbed. I was obsessed with horses, so we made it a point to check out the Kentucky Horse Park, and Chincoteague Island.

These trips were the high point of my boring suburban existence. As a child, I'd become thrilled with the idea of taking a two hour car trip to my cousins' house, simply because I knew I'd see new things. When I gained the freedom that comes with a driver's license and my own semi-reliable vehicle, things really took off. In college, I'd quietly creep off with a friend or two to check out any place that might be more exciting than the small town in which I lived- Chicago, Detroit, Pittsburgh.

You would think that being twenty something, postgraduate, with a brand new pile of bills to pay would have calmed down my urge to explore a bit, but I managed to land a fancy corporate job, and as my career flourished, so did my paychecks. I also came equipped with the standard responsibility level of a young college grad, which is to say I managed to keep myself and my cat alive, but the rest of my choices were somewhat questionable.

As a result, my bonuses and raises were spent on travel. I went to Boston, Baltimore, and Washington DC. My time off accrued as I put in long hours and late nights at the office, eking my way ahead in the corporate world, and I'd cheerfully fritter it all away by meeting up with friends and family all over the country.

Fast forward about ten years, and things couldn't be more different. I was still working for a large corporation, but now I had become completely disillusioned with the whole thing. My career had really taken off, but I hadn't had a vacation that hadn't been consumed with work in several years. Sure, I still travelled- in fact, I fell in love with hiking and backcountry excursions shortly after I met my husband Brad, but I also remained tied to my Blackberry in case I got an urgent client email. I even got a crisis call from a client while I was attending my grandmother's funeral. It was all too much for me.

After one weekend of backcountry and hiking, which had been unsurprisingly cut short by some payroll calculation crisis or another, I remember driving home thinking, "there's got to be another way." It's not that I hated my career, but I was angry at how much of me was devoted to answering phone calls, emails, and dealing with other people's problems, when all I wanted to do was stare off into a brand new horizon and let the amazing views, cultures, scenes and people of this planet sink into my soul.

That's when I saw it, puttering over the horizon towards us. It was old, and brown, but in pristine condition. I turned to Brad and said, "What if we dropped everything and lived in a VW bus?" Shockingly, he didn't drive off the road. I think he said something to the effect of "yeah, that would be cool." In the grand tradition of spouses everywhere, I think he was giving me about 45% of his attention.

Much to the astonishment of everyone privy to the plan, we turned the key in the ignition of our 1985 VW Vanagon about three years later. I can't say "and we never looked back," because there was a lot of second guessing, regret, fear, and tears that first year. If you've ever coasted down the highway during rush hour with a giant cloud of black, noxious smoke following you, you're probably familiar with the feeling of wanting to teleport yourself to another dimension, ASAP.

But, we stuck with it. Here we are, on the road, and while I'd love to say "since we were fabulously wealthy, we never had to work again," that would be a lie. Overall, our daily living expenses have dropped dramatically. We still enjoy eating, doing laundry, putting gas in the van, and the occasional hotel room when we find ourselves getting super grumpy about dirt, inclement weather, and especially bugs.

As with all of my books to date, what you're about to read comes from years of personal experience, including many experiments: some that failed miserably, and some that succeeded brilliantly. Both Brad and I work on the road, but we have very different types of jobs. He's still in the corporate space, sweating through twelve hour conference calls, while I'm a freelancer.

The question we field the most is whether we actually earn money? The answer is yes, of course. We're charitable people, but we do the work so we can get paid. We have bank accounts and expenses, just like everyone else. Our pay is set up as a direct deposit. Brad is paid bi-weekly, and I'm paid shortly after each deadline I meet.

This book will walk through many of the decisions and situations I and others who work from the road have had to consider along the way. While I will share my own experiences, the topics that I cover will be familiar to anyone who has made the transition from an office setting to WFH, remote worker, or telecommuter status. I've interviewed others who have gone from a traditional office setting to the view of their choice, and I have researched the advice of experts and those who have been doing this far longer than Brad and I have.

One thing to bear in mind is that every experience will be different. While Brad and I don't have children, for example, I've been sure to interview couples who are working on the road with families. In short, it would be impossible to be able to cover every "what if" scenario. Instead, I've chosen to write about some of the very common struggles, decisions, and considerations that many people have experienced when leaving the office behind to pursue the work environment of their dreams.

Next we'll take a look at why you might wish to follow in the footsteps of so many others and take your job away from the office environment. There are many minute details you'll want to consider. The goal of this book is to prepare you for those little bumps in the road before you encounter them.

Whether you're rethinking your decision to work on the run, or just starting to consider the possibilities, know that you are not alone, and that there is a practical solution for every situation that occurs!

## Chapter Two: Where Are You? An Exercise in Learning More About Yourself

If you're reading this book, then working from your home or anywhere outside the office is clearly on your mind. It might be the start of an idea, or you might be fully engaged in the process. Either way, you know your intention, but the road to success might not be as obvious as you hoped it would be.

The first hurdle that has to be cleared is purely psychological: WHY do you want to work remotely?

It may not feel like it yet, but this is actually a pretty big decision to make. Many things will change by leaving the office, and whether or not those changes feel beneficial or too difficult will depend greatly on your lifestyle, your attitude, and your overall mental state.

At this stage, you'll likely have a cloud of thoughts buzzing around your mind. Organization is the key. Whether you're the type who likes to jot lists or keep a journal, or the type who requires a linear system like swimlanes or an Excel spreadsheet, it's important to keep track of these thoughts. Like insects swarming a campfire, they'll quickly retreat, only to be replaced with new concerns and details.

So let's start by creating the first list or spreadsheet to answer the questions below :

>*How did you get here?*
>*Why do you want to work remotely?*

There may be a myriad of answers to these questions, but make sure to take the time to write them all down. No one else has to read this list or sheet, so you have nothing to hide. Include everything from the most major concerns ("I feel trapped in this lifestyle") all the way down to the petty ones ("There's never coffee left by the time I get to the office and I have to buy my own"). Everything that's on your mind is valid at this point. Don't fool yourself into thinking this is a simple black-and-white situation. Explore your list and consider what having your time and location to yourself can help you accomplish in the long run.

Many people have a hard time starting this exercise. There are so many thoughts and emotions that come to mind when considering the activities that take up most of your waking hours. It might help you to walk through your daily experience so you can identify pain points or things for which you are grateful on a step-by-step basis.

While everyone's office experience is a bit different, chances are that your day in the office looks something like this:

1. You wake up every morning to choose an outfit that meets someone else's dress code.

2. You drive through mind-bending traffic to the office building someone else has selected, sitting in a chair you don't like at the desk that has been assigned to you.

3. Your coworkers are decent enough, but you spend the majority of the day in the company of people you don't know, using equipment that dozens of others have used before you. Both you and the

equipment are assigned identification numbers, rather than having an actual identity.

4. The highlight of your days is usually taking breaks at the appointed times to escape to a limited number of places that can be accessed in the allotted span of the break. Alternately, you sit at your desk, checking out only the websites that the company firewall permits you to view, or trying to get a signal on your phone so you can take a quick peek at your social media or texts.

5. If all goes well, you are permitted to leave the office at the regularly scheduled hour, but sometimes you have to stay late to finish a task, work with a customer, or deal with piles of work. If you're paid on an hourly basis, you might enjoy the overtime pay, but if you're salaried, it may not be so exciting.

6. Then you get another mind-bending commute home, in which you attempt to relax and shake off the challenges and stress of the day, have a peaceful dinner, and get some sleep before it all repeats again the next day.

As you read this list, some or all of it may resonate with you. Alternatively, there may be some sections that don't speak to your experience. Naturally, this isn't going to be reflective of every person's specific situation, but the experience described above is common amongst those who work in an office building. What types of images or feelings come up as you read through this example? Where do those thoughts and emotions belong on the list or sheet you are creating?

For example, you might be feeling restricted and stifled as you read this list. You may feel that your workplace has too many rules and regulations. Maybe you feel there are too many decisions being made for you.

You may notice that in this example, there's very little flexibility for the incidental occurrences of daily life. This type of working model expects bodies in seats for a specific amount of time each day. So if you or a family member have an appointment, you'll likely have to take at least part of the day off, especially with travel time factored in. Depending on your company's time off policies, you may or may not get paid for that time away from your desk.

Time off might be hard to come by as well. While you may yearn to spend summer days at the beach with your family, that might also be the busy season for your business, which means watching the sunset from your desk, rather than from a gorgeous oceanfront.

If there's an accident or emergency, you've got to work things out with your job before you can give full attention to the situation. While many managers are understanding, a quick google search will reveal plenty of horror stories in which an incident that could have been resolved with a little sympathy results in the loss of a job... or worse.

One major draw towards working remotely is control. When you take your job offsite, you often gain control over much of your daily work experience. That can include everything from the hours that you work, to where you work, and when and how you spend your lunch hour.

Working remotely doesn't guarantee that you'll be able to breeze through every appointment, spend every day lounging at the beach, or ensure that nothing bad will ever happen. It just means that you'll have the ability to make minor adjustments based on your real-life needs, rather than spending a strict eight hours each day writhing under the control of your boss, your coworkers, or your customers. If you need a bathroom break, you can typically take one, instead of waiting for your scheduled-and-approved morning breaktime. If you need to drop your car off for an oil change during your lunch break, your boss can not tell you that you're not allowed to leave the premises until you clock out for the day.

You may find the idea of having this level of control very appealing. Rather than having to schedule time off for an appointment, you simply schedule your meetings and calls around that appointment. You mark the time as unavailable, and you make up the time by starting work earlier or working later. And instead of having to skip out on the family vacation year after year, perhaps you head down to the beach and watch the waves roll in as you field essential calls and emails.

Is it complete freedom? No, of course not. You still need to do the job you're getting paid to do. Your boss, Human Resources department, and overall corporate entity can still dictate the rules, and you still need to be crystal clear in all communication with coworkers and customers alike. But in this situation, working remotely gives you a greater level of control, from being able to take calls in your pyjamas, to logging in from a lounge chair.

Perhaps you want to take that even further. You don't just want to work from home- you want to work for yourself. Not everyone has to go the full nine yards like I did, leaving home and work behind to live in a van like a hippie and write all day. There are, however, many opportunities for those who wish to run a side-hustle or even a full-time gig from home or from the road. Predictably, many of these gigs offer even greater opportunities for control, and allow you to have almost complete flexibility over your hours as long as you are still completing any set projects and meeting your deadlines.

So, as you're making your list, lanes, spreadsheet, or idea map, keep these concepts in mind. You may find yourself starting to group your reasons into categories, such as "Things I Need to Control," or "Areas Where I Need Flexibility."

**Kristine's List**

For me, having control has always been a huge part of the decisions I've made, especially within my career. My transition from college to corporate life was pretty rough. I felt like I had to prove myself every single day. It wasn't unusual for me to work shifts of twelve hours or more, day after day after day. Ultimately, I was very successful in my role and made a huge impression on people at the executive level. But none of that saved me when the division I was working for was sold. The new company didn't have my role within their organizational structure, and since no one could figure out what to do with me, I was dismissed.

I was given a very healthy severance package with a huge financial incentive to stay "on call" for the remainder of the year. I did what most people who have suddenly had the rug pulled out from under them do. I made a series of irrational decisions that mostly involved not staying at home and moping. I traveled, hiked, and camped, distracting myself from putting any thought into the next steps of my career.

I could have saved myself a lot of time and trouble if I had paused for a moment and made a list of challenges, benefits, and sticking points, like the one you're working on right now. Instead, once my on call time ended, I took the first job that came my way, and started a career path through misery. If I had made a list, or even considered my career from a personal and emotional viewpoint, I would have understood what makes me tick. Instead, I was still feeling the pressure of impressing everyone, doing a good job, and putting in a deathly amount of effort to prove my worth. (And I do mean deathly- I ended up being hospitalized with a severe case of bronchitis that I stoically ignored while I was trying to master a particularly tricky job duty.)

The idea of writing out why you want to work from home and how you got to this potential decision may seem silly or feel awkward, but it's the sort of uncomfortable exercise we all need to visit from time to time to truly understand what's on our mind and in our hearts. If I had known during that tumultuous time what I know now, I would've saved myself a good ten years of stress, heartache, headaches, and anxiety. My list would have looked something like this:

Why do I want to work remotely?

- My work environment is distracting due to a gossiping coworker who simply will not stop coming to my cubicle to tell me I'm going to get fired for some randomly perceived transgression.
- Coming to work at 7.30am is dangerous due to security not being on site until 9am.
- Scheduling meetings with East Coast and West Coast clients means no lunch break or dinner break- I'm working 7:30am to 8pm every day.
- I literally have no clean clothes because there's no time to do laundry.
- Since my manager works in another state and time zone, why do I need to be onsite?
- Due to VPN and laptop access, many of my job duties can be completed from any location with internet access.
- I spend the entire day in meetings about scheduling meetings. I could dial in to these meetings or skip them entirely so that I can focus on client-based tasks that are more urgent and more valuable for the company's bottom line.
- I have actually started to cry during rush hour traffic because I just want to be at home, in my pyjamas, eating a sandwich, in bed before I pass out for three hours and do it all over again.

As you can see, some of these items are perfectly rational, such as not wanting to walk through an urban location in the dark without security guards present. Other line items are things I need to work through on my own, like not having clean laundry. Others still are very much emotionally driven, like crying in traffic about a sandwich.

All of these items are valid, though. Every single item on this list inspired a new form of stress for me, to the point where I was so distracted by hating this routine, that I could barely take a deep breath and focus long enough to think about my actual tasks needing to be done. I was filled with a boiling resentment for all the things I needed to accomplish but couldn't.

At first, my list would have just said something like, "Because I hate it here and my life is in shambles and I don't know what to do." Only in a screaming, hysterical voice, because that's where I was emotionally.

Making this list is going to help you understand why you dislike your current job situation and help you discover that maybe you don't hate everything, after all. Unpacking your complicated thoughts and emotions that are urging you to work off-site will help you understand if that's what you really want, or if you just need to make some other personal changes in your life.

Maybe working from home or remotely is the best decision for you, but perhaps you just need a new job altogether. You might just need to simply sit down with your boss to discuss scenarios like your distracting coworker. The first step to understanding where you're headed is to create a list that includes every one of your problems- from the very real to the incredibly petty- that is pushing you away from the standard 8 hour office environment.

## Chapter Three: The Pros & Cons of Working Remotely

After the previous exercise, you will likely be feeling one of three ways:
- More driven than ever to transition to working on the run
- Completely lost, confused, and possibly terrified
- Absolutely certain you'll never make this work

As someone who has made the transition myself, I will assure you that you will continue to feel these three waves of emotion throughout the rest of your career. Because there is absolutely no certainty in life, you can only do so much to prepare yourself for the endless barrage of "what ifs" that will surely come to surface. You'll at least be more aware of what you're looking at and have confidence in your ability to face the unknown.

The next step in preparing for a world far away from cubicles is identifying the pros and cons of working remotely. Again, these are not going to be the same for everyone and will probably be just as complicated as the first exercise. The overall goal of pinning down the benefits and challenges is to help you discover how truly plausible it is for you to work from another location. This will help you determine if you truly can use this method as an office escape.

To get you started, here are some of the most common pros and cons for working remotely sourced from my entire network of remote workers. This list encompasses freelancers, side-hustlers, crafters, and corporate telecommuters, and it is by no means reflective of every situation. This is just a little bit of inspiration to get you started on your own personal journey!

| Pros | Cons |
| --- | --- |
| I can work from literally any location with a Wifi signal | I've had to purchase/replace/service all of my own equipment |
| I don't have to spend two hours each day in my car | Sometimes I have to drop what I'm doing to go into the office for meetings/presentations |
| I don't have to change my lifestyle | I spend a lot more time on the phone than I did when I was in the office |
| Flexible hours- I log in when I want/need to | No social connection with my coworkers |
| Greater opportunities are available to me through freelancing | I have to discipline myself to complete all of my work on time |
| Since I'm not physically locked in meetings, I am more productive and present for my clients | My kids/pets think they need to sing or scream through every conference call |
| I get to spend more time with my family | Sometimes important information doesn't get to me, because it's discussed person-to-person in the office, and no one thinks to email me |
| I am far more productive without distractions | I have to be more creative and patient with myself when it comes to carving out time to work on very difficult/serious tasks |

As you write out and discover your own personal pros and cons list, consider the weight you give to each item. For example, being able to work from any place with a WiFi signal was the most significant detail on my own personal list, whereas having to deal with my own equipment barely registered as being a negative thing. I would list my semi-functioning equipment as a "mild irritant," rather than a full-out "con." For you, however, that might be a huge impediment.

The same goes for distractions. I like to joke that Brad could complete a formal presentation through a full-blown hurricane, whereas I've been known to lose an entire hour because a butterfly landed on my hand. When you're working on your own, there will be both hurricanes and butterflies, on a literal and metaphorical level. Are you disciplined enough to keep yourself on track no matter what? Furthermore, is your job forgiving of these interruptions? For me, as a freelancer, I can simply add extra hours at the end of my day as needed, or continue writing a draft in a notebook. Brad, on the other hand, has to race to the nearest free WiFi spot any time our signal is interrupted, so that he can stay connected.

Your lifestyle is going to determine a lot of the pros and cons of working remotely. If part of the reason you're planning to change up your job situation is because your lifestyle is about to become radically different, add that to your pros and cons list, too.

In my situation, I had quit my job and lived on the road for quite some time before I started thinking about a new job. In that time, I did a lot of thinking about what I was going to do, and how I was going to make it work. Since my first transition, in which I put absolutely no thought into what I was doing, didn't turn out so well, I decided to put a lot of conscious effort into my new job. I did these exact exercises that I'm recommending to you now. In my experience, you can absolutely jump in the water and see if you can figure out how to swim before you drown, or you can learn about the mechanics of swimming before you approach the shoreline and give yourself a fighting chance of floating on safely.

## Chapter Four: What Will You Accomplish With This Change?

There is one thing you need to know before we go any further with these exercises. You may still be thinking that working from home, the road, or your beachfront dreamhouse will allow you many hours of staring off dreamily into the distance. Perhaps you'll gain some time to do that, but let me assure you now:

**If you want to slack off, this is not the workstyle for you.**

No matter how hard you work in the office, you will still spend time taking breaks, chatting with coworkers, lingering over the coffee machine, walking up and down aisles to stimulate thoughts, having post-meeting rap sessions, and more. It's simply part of the office experience.

When you work from home, the stakes are higher, and the pressure is on. You are still expected to be on your A-game all day, but now there are distractions like you have never encountered before. Instead of having a walk-and-talk meeting to grab a cup of coffee with your manager, you'll find yourself walking with your laptop to the coffee maker so that you can continue your Skype conversation while you pour yourself that second cup of coffee you have desperately craved for the past two hours. Instead of dashing into the bathroom to check your appearance before an important meeting, you'll find yourself lecturing anyone who shares your home on the importance of staying completely quiet, even if there is an emergency, all while trying to coax your printer to unjam, and fielding a call from your coworker, who wants to know if you received the email she needs you to print out before the meeting.

It is very common for those who work outside of the office to report higher productivity, a greater focus on their work, and an unbelievable amount of output compared to when they had worked in the office. The difference, many hypothesize, is due to the level of discipline that we exercise when working from home, a van, a coffee shop, or our beachfront dream home.

At work, it's easy to give into distractions, because they're either tangentially work-related (that walk-and-talk to the coffee maker, for example), or they're your reward for doing something difficult (treating yourself to a sandwich from your favorite deli because you finished a report early, perhaps). Either way, any time you are in the office but not doing work, you still feel a sense that what you're doing is relevant to your job, and thus, you deserve to get paid for it.

It is extremely difficult to feel justified in getting paid for watching a butterfly sit on your hand for twenty minutes while you upload pictures of it to Instagram. You will absolutely feel more alive and connected to this planet, but if your boss or client asks why you dropped off a meeting abruptly, they are not going to be amused by butterfly pictures.

Perhaps there's a layer of guilt that drives those of us who work from our ideal location. Some say that expectations of remote workers are higher, because the jealous parties still in the office are hoping they'll fail. Likely, it's a little bit of both, along with the freedom from that burning anger or hopelessness that you felt in the office. Having more control and being at peace can be a miracle elixir for improving productivity.

The key part of that phrase, however, is "CAN BE." You know yourself better than anyone else. You know what you're capable of. You know how many mountains you can comfortably move each day. You know how much your kids, pets, partner, surroundings, etc., will distract you.

In the next section of this book, we'll look at the different types of jobs that translate well to working remotely and working on the run. If you're thinking, "I can definitely handle the lifestyle, but not with my current job," then stick with this. We'll get there.

Maybe the opposite is true, and your current thoughts are, "Sure, my job would be ideal to take on the road, but I'm not sure I can wrap my head around stepping out of an office." No worries- there's a section for that too. Alternately, you might see the benefits and the possibilities, but the practicalities are way beyond your imagination. We'll definitely address those challenges, as well.

Before you put the effort into setting up a home office, before you hand in your resignation and take to the road, and before you admit out loud that you're interested in exploring the possibilities, you have to be real with yourself about your needs and what you want to get out of the experience.

I actually loved the job I quit in order to live on the road. I worked with a small group of people, and we loved each other like family. When I formally resigned, I used the phrase "it's not you; it's me" when talking to my boss. And while we laughed as I said it, it was true. I was not physically, mentally, emotionally, or psychologically intended to work from 8am to 5pm, Monday through Friday, regardless of what my work history indicated. Instead, I was born to work from when I get started to when I finish, 365 days a year.

Brad loves working. Brad loves working a little too much. While I might need an entire day to pause and refresh my brain, he doesn't turn off. When he worked at the office, I would have to call him around 8 or 9pm to remind him to come home. That's because when he's fully accessible to his staff and coworkers, he gets sucked into every single task that comes his way. I have seen him listen in on one meeting with his phone while being physically present in another meeting. Now that he works on the road, his focus is crystal clear. Sure, people still reach out to him 24 hours a day, but people can't appear in his space to distract him. He has become far more productive in far fewer hours.

I mention this to illustrate that there are many different ways in which taking your job on the road- even if it's just to your own home- can be an extraordinarily beneficial move. We'll go into this in more detail in a later section, but if you have spent the majority of your career working in an office, you will make a series of discoveries about yourself, your working method, your patience level, and more as you transition out of the office and into a solitary work style. The exercises I provide in this book are meant to gently ease you into this new reality, so that you don't find yourself in just as chaotic a situation as you found in the office.

Working from a location of your choice can help you control cost of living by allowing you to work in the town, state, country, or 1985 Volkswagen Vanagon of your choice. To a certain extent, working remotely gives you the opportunity to have full control over your work schedule, and what you accomplish in any given 24 hour period. You'll even have the ability to finally define what your time and your money mean to you, which will set you on the path to your ultimate career goals.

At the same time, acting upon this decision will require a great deal of discipline. You will face some uncomfortable truths about yourself. You will cry, you will fail, and you will have many awkward learning moments along the way. But, if you're willing to pick yourself up, dust yourself off, and head back to the drawing board a few times, armed with some constructive criticism and advice, you may be on the first leg of your journey to the work/life balance you've always dreamed of.

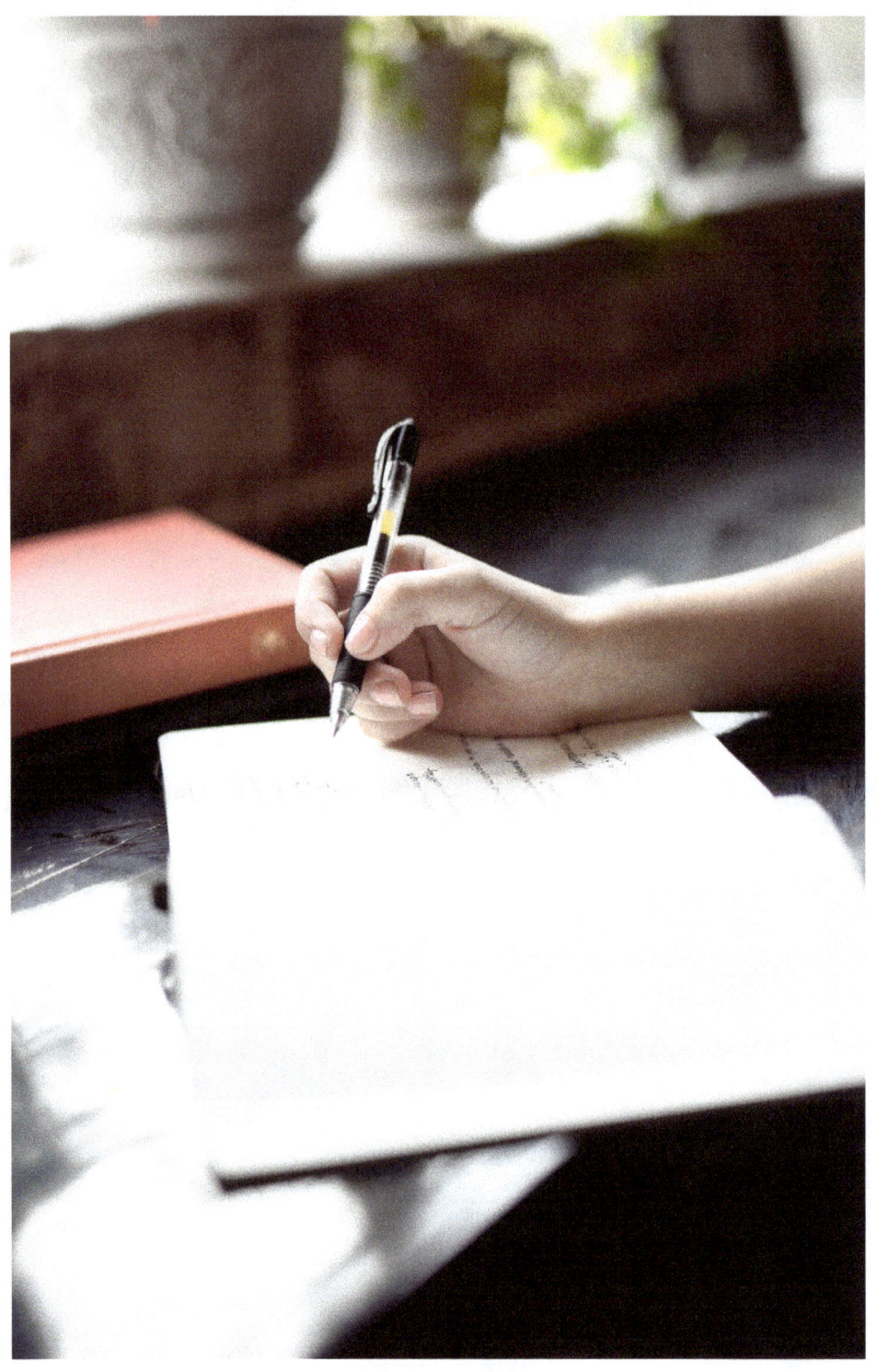

## Section Two: Details, Details, Details

In the first section, we focused on exercises that will help wrap your brain around the why of wanting to take your work away from the office. Hopefully, that helped clarify some of the thoughts, emotions, and noise that has been buzzing around in your brain whenever you think about the topic of your career.

Now, you might be dealing with a different kind of buzzing: that of what your job is actually going to look like once you head out on your own. Are you interested in maintaining your current position, or something similar to it? Or are you ready to strike out on your own in a whole new area of expertise such as a freelancer, crafter, or hired hand? What types of skills are you willing to tap into, equipped to exercise, and can translate to the environment in which you're planning to work?

This is the time for hashing out details, and with that will come both answers to some of your current concerns, as well as a whole new batch of questions. Rest assured, that this book is intended to put you in the right position to answer all of those questions, even those which are exclusive to your current situation.

## Chapter One: Determining the Who, Where, When, and How of Working on the Run

You are now in the Preliminary Stage of transitioning out of the office environment. This is the time to gather your resources and figure out what you want to do when you grow up, and how you plan to get to that point from here.

This journey may take a lot of directions. So far, you may not have considered the possibilities of a new job. As mentioned earlier, you might be perfectly happy with your current job and are willing to do what it takes to work with your employer to maintain the status quo, even if you're not physically present in the main office at all times.

Alternatively, you may have read the phrase "what you want to be when you grow up" and felt a spark of something inside. Maybe there's a certain inspiration that this transition could be a really big deal for you, as you finally go after that dream you've been harboring since you were a small child.

Anything is possible at this point in time, and it's up to you to decide what type of journey you're going to take here. In fact, it's time for another soul-searching, brainstorming session.

For this exercise, you might need a pen and some paper. You are going to go deep here, and ask yourself the one question that's going to set up the success of your transition from the office to the world. I recommend finding a quiet area, where you'll have minimal distractions and plenty of thinking space.

**Your Challenge: An Exercise in Reality**
The focus of this session is logistics: **How do you think this is going to work?** What comes to mind when you sit down and really think about working from the home, on the run, or anywhere in between?

Brad and I completed this exercise at different times, and our responses couldn't have been more different.

Brad actually started telecommuting about five years before we bought the van. Through a variety of job transitions, he found himself faced with the option to either move to Colorado, or start working from home. At the time, his family was a huge factor in our decision not to move, so he opted to set up a desk in the corner of our exercise room and started the process that way.

For Brad, there was little in the way of making the decision. Once he announced his plan to work from home, his company provided him with all of the equipment and technology necessary to move forward. They even sent him a fun desk organizer to congratulate him on his choice. His transition from working at home to van life was a bit more involved, but we'll cover that in more detail in the next section.

On the flip side, I had much more time to think about it, since I went from working full time in an office to living in a van with no transition. I started my journey of working on the run by daydreaming. In fact, I personally worked on this exercise a lot at night, staring up at the mosquito-speckled roof of the van, trying to quiet the panic that was rapidly rising every time I thought about "working" or "jobs."

I was equipped with a Creative Writing degree with the majority of my resume including writing as well. Ever since I was a child, the only thing I had really wanted to do was write, and I'd considered myself incredibly lucky that I had had multiple opportunities to flex that particular muscle throughout my seemingly-unrelated career in HR/Benefits and insurance. In fact, I'd gone on to pursue post-graduate certifications in various types of communications and marketing, so that I could do more writing, regardless of the position I held at the moment.

When I started daydreaming, I kept coming back to "what if I could write for a living?" So, on my mental map, I made that the start and end of all of my decision making. I was going to write. Now what I was going to write and how I was going to find gigs were beyond me at this stage, and getting paid was a mystery that I hoped to solve sooner rather than later, but I had made up my mind.

Brad's and my situations represent just two of the ways you can look at this particular brainstorming session. You can stick with what you know, or you can go directly to manifesting your wildest dreams.

A visualization exercise is best for this quandary. Close your eyes, and picture yourself working. Are you seated at a laptop? Are you physically creating something? Are you in a quiet room, a noisy cafe, or surrounded by nature? What are your hands doing? What are your eyes looking at? Most importantly, how do you feel?

You're looking for a visual or daydream that makes you feel peaceful, alive, and productive. While there is not a single job I can think of that doesn't result in some form of cursing and wanting to throw everything out the window, that should not be the standard. In fact, for many, that's the reason you're completing this exercise in the first place.

So again, what does your new career look like? Is it the same thing, only in a different place? Or is it a brand new opportunity with horizons you haven't even begun to explore yet?

If these cerebral activities are starting to wear on you, I have good news: the next few exercises in this chapter are going to be purely objective. The next round of lists and brainstorming will be strictly fact-based, designed to help you manifest the reality that you just conjured in your visualizations.

## Chapter Two: Who, Where, and When- Just the Facts

Even if you plan on doing this alone, know that you aren't really alone. You may be one person in an apartment, bungalow, van, skoolie, or yurt, but no one can have a career without someone to pay them.

That means you have to identify your connections and your network. If your aim is to continue your current job outside of the regular work boundaries, then your network will be fairly simple to identify. List everyone you require to make your job work. This can include:
- Your manager/supervisor
- Any superiors with whom you work directly on a regular basis
- Admins/support staff
- Schedulers
- Coworkers with whom you share projects or common duties
- IT/Tech Support
- Human Resources
- Benefits Helpline/ Employee Resource Center

You may also choose to reach out to others who work from home or telecommute that perform similar jobs to yours. They can act as mentors or at least springboards for any questions and thoughts you might have as your life quickly changes.

If you are going to continue to work your current job from a different location, you want to align yourself with connections that will help foster your productivity and keep you in touch with things that are happening inside the office. That can include anything from the latest water cooler discussions, to office gossip, or any underground rumblings about upcoming changes and projects.

For those who are thinking of spreading their wings elsewhere, you may already be feeling a little anxious about your network. First of all, know that you are not alone, either. When I started to feel drawn to a life of freelancing on the road, I lamented to Brad that I didn't know anyone who did this, and no one would ever understand me. As dramatic as that sounds, it felt like the truth to me. Going from a highly-structured corporate environment with timed bathroom breaks to a world where I simply have to deliver a quality product by a certain date is about as polar opposite as you can get in the working world. My friends— and even Brad— get second-hand anxiety when I tell them I took an afternoon nap, or that I ditched my manuscript for an early morning hike. It really seems like no one understands freelancers except for other freelancers.

Know that you are not alone. You are not the only person working on their own terms. Anyone who has a side-hustle, a personal business, or even someone who occasionally sells their creative works knows what you're going through. It doesn't have to be their full-time passion in order for them to appreciate your experience. These people are helpful connections.

So when you're making this list of your connections, be sure to include:
- People who own or have owned their own business
- Your friend who retired from corporate but now does pet portraits by commission only
- That person in the office who makes and sells soaps and lotions

- The person whom you've loosely connected to on social media who does freelance accounting
- Your nephew who makes several hundred bucks a month pet sitting
- Your chef friend who offers meal planning advice
- That guy you met at a bar who lives in a van and has the coolest Instagram ever

While your exact examples will surely differ, this group is about to become your biggest support network. Anyone who works independently with clients is going to be a wealth of information as you discover how to market yourself and your abilities. They may not understand all the elements of your particular situation, but these will be the people you call on when you need advice. When you suspect a client is trying to underpay you, you'll know who to contact. When you can't get a Wi-Fi signal even though everything is set up according to instructions, you'll know where to send a message for immediate help. If you're looking for an accountability buddy to prevent you from chasing butterflies for a few hours, these are the people who will know exactly what you mean by that and can coach you through a little self-discipline.

Now that you have your virtual team lined up, you need to size up the playing field. Location and surroundings have an incredible impact on anyone's ability to be productive and successful. The stress of the office environment might be one reason you're pursuing this option in the first place!

You will need to make sure that you have a designated work area, which we'll discuss in more detail later on. But for now, consider the following questions:
- Where will I work?
- Do I have adequate access to Wi-Fi, electricity, a phone signal, etc in this location?

If the answer to your first question is "in my home office," then you'll have no trouble with the second question. But if the answer to your first question is anything like mine- "in my van"- then the second question is answered with a solid "maybe?"

Those who are planning to truly work on the run need to strategize. Does your van/skoolie/RV have an adequate generator? Do you have decent Wi-Fi service nearly everywhere? Can you use your phone as a hotspot in an emergency?

In our case, Brad attends meetings almost all day, so he needs to have access to continuous phone signal and Wi-Fi. We have to be extremely strategic about staying "city-side" long enough for him to complete a work day, before we head out into the backcountry, where there might not be any sort of signal.

For many of us Van Lifers, this is a huge sacrifice, because we desperately want to be offline, off the grid, and somewhere wild and unrecognizable. If you haven't had the opportunity to drive across America, you may be surprised at how much of this country is completely un-wired. It's a beautiful sensation... until you can't send a client that file that's due at 9pm EST, you get dropped off of a phone call six times in a row, or you lose all of your edits because you didn't put your document on the cloud before you fell off the grid.

This is, unfortunately, the reality of working on the run. Though you want to be far from everything, there are some ties to the so-called "real world" that just cannot be severed. They can, however, be minimized by carefully selecting your location and being very deliberate in your scheduling.

This brings us to the "when" of working remotely. Regardless of whether your "where" is a spare bedroom or a converted school bus, you're going to need to know when you're working. Many people who leave the office find themselves working 24 hours, 7 days a week, 365 days per year. For the majority of the people who work this schedule, it is highly undesirable. It is an easy trap to fall into when you're not working in an office. Imagine you are knee-deep in a work project. As you type along, you don't notice the hours fly by, because you're completely engrossed. It's Thursday night, none of your programs are on. At some point, you stuff some cheese and crackers in your face because your stomach rumbles, but you keep working. There are no interruptions. Everything is great. Suddenly, you notice it's dark, so you glance down at the tiny clock on the bottom of your screen. 11:59pm. Seriously?

Pulling an all-nighter or an extra-long shift isn't unheard of in any industry. But it can easily become a habit when you don't have that social signal to get up, power down the computer, and go home. Your chair is cozy, your room is familiar, and all of the food and drinks you need are just a few steps away. While this can work for an extremely busy day, be careful about letting this become your usual schedule.

Humans need "on" time and "off" time. If your brain is constantly in performance mode, you will burn out very, very quickly. You will fail to enjoy anything that's going on around you, mostly because you don't notice it's happening. Your boss and team will come to expect you to be available 24/7, and you will resent them for this expectation. Work will become your life. Worst of all, you will potentially alienate everyone around you because you have made work your top priority and have placed everything else on the back burner.

I was headed down that path myself. When I first started freelancing, it was all too easy for me to work all of the time. I found myself getting up at 5am to start projects so I could have them submitted the same day. Unfortunately, my creative muses didn't appreciate this enthusiasm, and after a few weeks, I found myself completely unable to write. Words started looking strange. Amazingly, this confusion and extreme writer's block cleared up completely once I took a nice long nap, allowed myself some deep breaths and generous exercise, and took the opportunity to consume a few nutritious meals with the laptop closed.

Therefore, I strongly recommend that you exercise that control that you so crave by creating a schedule, even if you are not in a physical office. In the very first exercise of this book, we identified some of the reasons you wanted to work from home, and I mentioned that for nearly everyone, having control over your time and location is the number one factor. Now it is time to put that autonomy into effect.

Based on your sleeping habits, working through the night might be the best option for you. Or, if you have a lot of stuff to attend to, perhaps you schedule an "appointment day," where you allow yourself a few hours of time to take care of business, and make up those hours on other days. This can be extremely helpful for staying organized, since you'll know that any appointments you make will happen during that specific window of time, say, 8am to noon every Thursday. But best of all with this flexibility, you can take care of your own personal needs and develop your day around them.

Take a look at our schedules as examples of how this can work for you:

| Brad | Kristine |
| --- | --- |
| Wake: Between 8am and 9am MST Immediately exercise a bit | Wake: At exactly 6:04am EST each morning<br>Immediately exercise a bit |
| 9:00am-10:00am: Make coffee, read emails, review previous day's projects | 6.30am-10.30am: Organize files for the day and begin work |
| 10:00am-2:00pm: Meetings, work, phone calls | 10.30am-12:00pm: Eat and nap |
| 2:00pm: Lunch | 12:00pm-5:00pm: Continue Working |
| 2:15pm forward: Continue working until falling asleep. | 5:00-6:00pm: Close the laptop and call it a day. |

There are, of course, exceptions to these schedules but generally speaking, this is what we adhere to. Brad's home office is on Mountain Standard Time, so he works on their schedule, regardless of where we are. None of my clients are in the same time zone, so I keep myself on Eastern Standard Time sheerly out of habit. Brad doesn't work on Saturday and Sunday, while I do, but typically only part of the day. Brad never sets an alarm, but I wake up to the same annoying noise every day at exactly the same time. These schedules are simply reflections of how we operate as people. I need something to get me up and motivated in the morning, or I'll stay in bed all day. I also need to specifically turn off by a set time, while Brad keeps going until he reaches a decent stopping point.

Looking at these schedules, which is more attractive to you? What is most reasonable for your job and work style? Do you have to be near a phone at specific times? Do you have tasks that need to be completed by a strict deadline? Are you a self-motivated kind of person, or do you drizzle your way from task to task as the mood strikes?

Again, some of these are pretty philosophical questions, and you'll most likely find yourself changing your mind a few times as you try to hit your stride. Early in my freelancing career, I received an email from an angry client who was perturbed that I didn't answer her Skype calls at 3am. "Aren't your type supposed to be up and available all hours of the day?" she asked. I spent a significant amount of time wondering if I should be. After all, this was my career of choice; shouldn't I live up to the standards of my job? Ultimately, I decided the care of my own mental, physical, and emotional health— all of the things that I took into consideration when I transitioned out of the office and on my own— were more important than answering emails at 3am, so I simply replied, "I am available between 8am and 6pm, EST." And with a few exceptions, that has been true ever since. EST." And with a few exceptions, that has been true ever since.

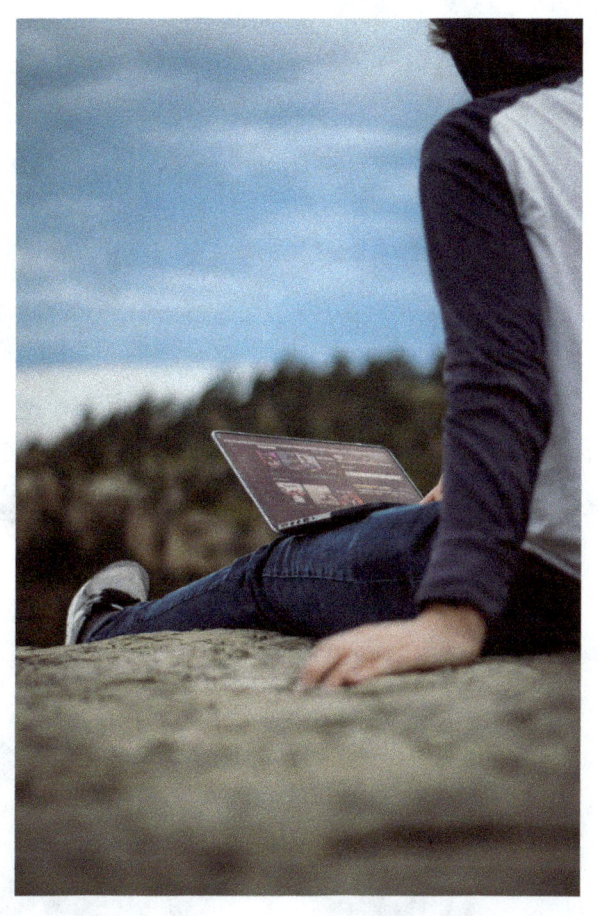

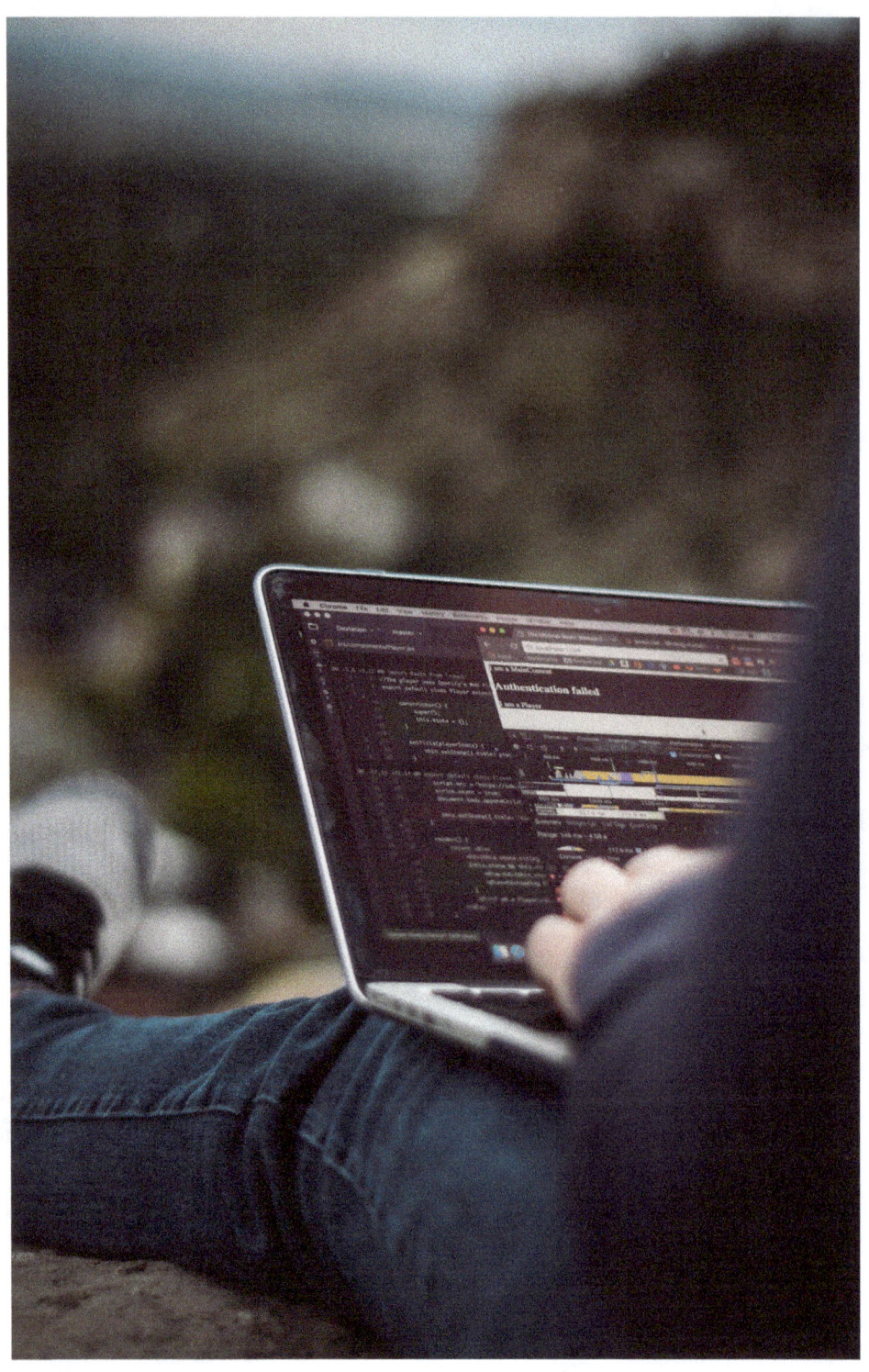

## Section Three: What Will I Be? What Will I Do?

So far, we've focused a lot on logistics. For some of you, this means that you're feeling more focused than ever, with a renewed sense of resolve to make this whole thing happen. Others still might feel a lot of apprehension, with thoughts such as, "It's great that I know my support network, but I don't even know what my job is going to be, or if I'm going to be able to afford to live!"

Those are valid concerns. Here's the thing when it comes to changing your lifestyle completely: It can be done immediately, but you will feel so much more prepared if you have taken the time to reflect on your resources, your needs, and your goals. When my division was sold, and I found myself suddenly jobless, one of the most uttered phrases at the resulting "Unhappy Hours" was "I just wish I'd been prepared." This is your chance to make a bid for greatness. Assuming you aren't already in a jobless position, you have all the opportunity you need to get your ducks in a row first.

Or maybe you have already been let go, or in an inspired moment, told your boss you're going to go live in a van. I've been there, as well. There are a lot of ways we can get to this point- some are positive, and some are not so pleasant. Some of you are about to be the happiest you've ever been. Even more of you are going to use this experience as a springboard to something more amazing than ever.

In this section, we're going to look at different jobs, and put them to the "on the run" test. There are some jobs that make absolutely no sense as WFH or van life jobs. However, if that is your field, you can still make this van lifestyle work.

The next several chapters are going to introduce various opportunities. Some of them may not feel as if they are relevant to your specific situation, but I encourage you to read the chapter anyway (or at least give it a healthy skim). There will be some tips, words of wisdom, and things anyone can consider in each section.

## Chapter One: Same as It Ever Was

Brad loves his job. What he actually does is very technical and involved, but essentially, he provides support and client interfacing in software development for a global firm. Brad has always loved his job, and it shows. He is available 24/7, phone signal permitting. Brad once gazed across a canyon, observing the beauty of Bandelier National Monument while chatting about eligibility files with his team. He is dedicated to his job at a level that I personally consider unhealthy, but his job brings him great joy, so this works for him.

Brad's original plan was to quit his job. He had already been working from home, but we both agreed that it would be hard to live in a van with no plan or itinerary, while balancing an intensive full time job. So he gathered his management team, and calmly explained to them that he and his wife had decided they needed to live in a 1985 Volkswagen Vanagon and that he wanted to leave by this date. He let them know that they would need to carve out an exit strategy.

I wasn't there for the phone call, or the rest of the afternoon, but I was very anxious to hear how it went. Brad seemed off when he came downstairs at the end of the day, but I couldn't put my finger on what was wrong. He explained that his management team had told him that they really needed him, and after spending the day consulting with various corporate leaders, they had offered him a six month leave of absence with benefits, as well as a bonus if he returned to work on a specific date.

I personally love telling this story, because it goes to show that this type of job transition doesn't have to be a negative thing. You may be greatly surprised by how accommodating your employer is, if you approach the potential movement of your work space from a very practical and positive space.

When having these types of discussions with others in your workplace, it is beneficial for everyone involved if you are organized and have taken the time to prepare with a few notes about your own needs and goals identified.

We touched earlier on productivity, which is often at the forefront of every manager's mind. For the most part, the location of your actual body doesn't matter to your team so much as that you are actively working, meeting deadlines, and getting the job done. Therefore, before you start discussions with your boss, I encourage you to explore this topic with yourself, and to do so very honestly. It's easy to say "sure, I'm productive!" Take a look at all of your notepads in the office. Are they filled with work-related notes and productive efforts, or are they more grocery lists, calculations for your own bills, daydreams, and things that demonstrate you're not really attending meetings on a mental level? Reflect on your performance reports. Do they advise you to look into time management courses?

If self-discipline, motivation, and staying on task aren't your most valuable skill set, that's okay. In fact, many people find that working from home removes a lot of distractions. For example, you won't be able to wander the aisles of your office, looking for someone who wants to chat. You won't be tempted to walk down to the cafeteria for a superfluous cup of coffee because there are no sympathetic cafe workers for you to laugh and joke with, rather than hurrying back to the office.

Then again, maybe it's not the people that are the distraction. Maybe you're so done with your coworkers that you spend most of the day listening to music. If anyone knew how much time you spent looking up lyrics and re-playing sick drops, they'd probably take your audio card away, but as far as anyone can tell, you're over there typing away. Or it could be your phone and the world of social media that has you grasped in its talons of constant conflict and gossip. Will these temptations intensify when you work from a place where you can have constant access to anything you want?

For most people, that's not a situation they can accurately predict. You need to be able to critically look at your work style and identify HOW you get things done. Then you need to plan some actions that will help you with your focus, so that you can be productive.

I have always been a procrastinator. I'm famous for coming in with that eleventh hour Hail Mary for the win when it came to huge projects in the corporate setting. At the same time, I have always shown up, ready to work, and never neglected even the most trivial daily duties, like watering the office plants. This is why I get up so early. At 6:04am, hardly anyone in my network is posting on social media. My European friends are at work. My Australian and Asian buddies are ending their days, and no one else in my hemisphere is awake to text and chat with me. Brad is still asleep, so I can't torment him. The most distracting thing that happens in the morning is each glorious sunrise (weather permitting), and I absolutely allow myself a few quiet moments to enjoy that part of the day.

Generally speaking, though, that sets me up for a productive day. By the time Brad is awake and encroaching on my coffee supply, I'm already in work mode. There have been times I've had to hide my phone from myself. Sometimes I put on headphones and listen to binaural tones, because if I listen to anything with lyrics and a beat, I'm going to have a personal dance party. You have to know yourself so that you can figure out what needs to be done to rein yourself in.

Ask yourself a series of questions:

1. What is my go-to distractor? This could be social media, games on your phone, music, etc.

2. What is it that this distraction gives me? Perhaps it's social interaction, or maybe a mental break.

3. What happens if I try a more productive type of break? Consider closing your eyes and taking ten deep breaths, or getting up from your workstation, having a few sips of water, and returning. Sometimes you really do need to tune out for a minute, to refocus.

This confidence in your productivity is what will project to your manager and Human Resources team. In your early conversations, don't let productivity be an elephant in the room. Empathize with their concerns and demonstrate that you have already considered this, and that you've already taken measures to address this possible challenge.

Hand-in-hand with productivity comes practicality. Specifically, will you be available for the amount of time your job needs you, and within the typical working day? In some situations, such as the example mentioned earlier in which you need to make regular appointments, the hours you work will definitely need to change. This could be due to any number of things, including needing to drop kids off at school or daycare at a certain time, medical appointments, or even a reduction in weekly hours for your physical or mental health, etc.

Your employer is likely going to be concerned that you won't be able to meet deadlines adequately. Think of ways you can be transparent with your manager early on so that this is less of a worry. As time goes by, you'll prove through your actions that you're still productive and efficient, but at first, your team will worry that you're out there chasing butterflies with people like me, instead of getting work done. You can offer to create a project list, or use a time-tracking software to help put them at ease. It might make you feel micromanaged, but if you're focused and determined, there's really nothing to fear.

When discussing this with your employer, make sure you approach it through the lens of collaboration. Let your team know that you appreciate that this is going to be a huge change for your office group as well as yourself. Think of things you can do to ease the burden for all of you, and bring those up in your talks with your manager. Let your employer know your specific availability, and actually plan to show up at those times.

Employers want to know that you are going to be just as valuable when you aren't under their watchful gaze. Consider—and then share with them—your thoughts on the practicality of working off-site. If there is a particular job duty that would be a fantastic opportunity for your skillset offsite, bring that up, as well.

For example, in one client relationship management position, our group had to run a specific report for all clients each Friday. This report was massive and, because it included so much information, would lock up your laptop for hours, which essentially rendered you useless for completing any other tasks—including speaking to clients. Coincidentally, anyone who didn't have major meetings on Fridays was permitted to work from home. One Friday, as I was wrapping things up in my at-home office, I offered to run the report. Imagine how many lightbulbs went on with my team when I was able to send everyone the report results after a few hours, and no one lost productivity (in fact, I got a load of laundry done and started dinner). From then on, the report was run as the last task of the day by someone who was working from home.

This is the sort of innovation that can make the concept of working outside of the office look very appealing to all parties involved. Sure, you may have to take on a regular task that was previously shared, but as a compromise, you're also getting the freedom to work from anywhere, with the added bonus of a more flexible schedule.

Once you have your working hours settled, and your team has discussed a practical and reasonable approach to meeting all of your regular deadlines and maintaining productivity levels, it's time to get into the less subjective details.

The first thing to get out of the way is who is paying for what expenses. In many cases, your company will set you up with a laptop and other equipment. Depending on your industry, they might want the laptop to have certain specifications, drivers, and programs, which they'll want to install through internal tech support. You'll need to think about monitors, printers, a mouse, a keyboard, and any other supplies you deem necessary.

You'll also want to look into options regarding your telephone. Depending on your job, an employer will provide you with a specific phone to be used strictly for work purposes. Other employers are willing to foot your entire monthly phone bill or at least part of it if you use it for work. Many larger corporations have access to discounts from major cell phone providers, so this tends to work out well for everyone involved.

As you iron out these technological details, make sure you know where your tech support will come from. It's easy enough to jog down to IT to ask a quick question or to get more batteries for your mouse now, but when you're not working in the office, who do you call? Who pays for the batteries? Furthermore, does that company-issued cell phone have service where you're headed? If you have a problem with the phone, do you head to the provider's local retail shop, or call someone within your company? Knowing these things before they happen in the mountains of Idaho or somewhere deep within the Ozarks is crucial.

One sensitive subject that needs to be addressed is your total compensation package. If you're receiving benefits such as medical, dental, and vision insurance now, are those benefits contingent on the number of hours worked or on your work location? If so, what options are available for you to continue those benefits? Are you still eligible for time off if you're not physically in the office? That can include time off due to illness or injury, as well as any vacation time. Will you still accrue or receive time off allowances at the same rate? What about disability pay?

Another concern may be job protection under the Family Medical Leave Act (FMLA) or state-mandated leaves, such as maternity and paternity leaves. If part of the reason you're changing your job situation is to care for yourself or a family member who has medical needs, you'll definitely want to be sure that those types of protection are still extended to you if you work remotely.

At first, you might think that it will be simple to just pick up your job and move it to your house, your van, or any place you might prefer to work. However, once you start thinking more about logistics, you'll discover there's a lot more to it than the location of your laptop. Having open and frank discussions with your management team and Human Resources department will help you think about all the minutiae that are often taken for granted in an office environment.

Still, this is not an impossible task. Start by focusing on the main topics of productivity, practicality, and the day-to-day details. At first you may have to make compromises which benefit the company. Try hard to keep an open mind and appreciate the concerns your employer may have. Understand who you are as a worker, but also how you fit into the organization as a resource. You may fear that your manager doesn't "trust" you, but ultimately, the concerns they may have about your productivity and the practical aspects of your transition off-site are less personal, and more about the organization as a whole. Let them know you plan to be there 100 percent in mind and effort, just not in body, and the conversation will certainly be more positive.

## Chapter Two: Redefining the "Free" in "Freelancing"

For some reason, when most people think about freelancing, they immediately think of writing, journalism, and photography. That's not entirely incorrect; in fact, those are the most popular outlets of freelancing. However, contract work and consulting is available in all sorts of fields. Whether those positions are something you can incorporate into your lifestyle, though, is something you'll have to fully explore before you commit time or money.

For someone who lives in a van, I'm incredibly risk-averse. I enter the literal and proverbial water one toe at a time, and when I started considering the possibilities of freelance copywriting, I approached it very, very slowly. I started with lots of research. Every time Brad was behind the wheel, I would look up various temporary writing gigs. I read everything I could on the topic, from online magazine articles, to Reddit postings from people who currently freelance. I wanted to know what the experience was like before I jumped in.

Most people will find that this is a good move, because expectations and reality are rarely aligned when you first start working on your own. You will need to establish personal boundaries, but you need to make sure that the hard lines you draw are reasonable for what you want to do. When I implemented my strict availability guidelines, for example, I made myself ineligible for a lot of great gigs that would have been perfect for me... if I was willing to work until I literally keeled over. There will be a lot of situations in which you will have to uncomfortably say "no," but in each of these scenarios, it's necessary to do so.

So I urge you to start the freelance job hunt slowly and methodically. Read the horror stories. Look at the job postings. Don't get sucked in by the ads that promise you'll make six figures a year doing what you love. You can, of course, if you spend all of your time working, but van lifers especially don't like that concept. From the statistics to the anecdotes, read it all.

Then it's time to get to work on organizing yourself.

First, think about your talents and skill sets. What can you do that is marketable? Nearly everything can be turned into a freelance gig. I know accountants, dietary consultants, illustrators, videographers, photographers, personal assistants, telemedicine nurses and therapists, lifestyle and health coaches, and travel agents, all of whom can take their job wherever they care to be at any given time. If you need help getting ideas, take a look at popular freelance networking sites, like Fiverr or Upwork. Look at the different categories and postings, and get an idea where your niche is.

Next, look at the time you want to dedicate to these opportunities. If working a regular eight-hour workday is something you hope to continue, then go for it. If you want to have your days free, then work at night. For most gigs, the actual timing within the day doesn't matter as much as meeting deadlines and being available to communicate. Other gigs have specific time-related requirements. For example, photographers require a certain amount of light in order to shoot properly, and personal assistants need to be on the ball with deadlines.

Equipment is also an important thing to factor into this decision. If you're going to be sending lots of files, you'll want to make sure that your computer can handle a lot of data, and/or cloud access. If you're going to be creating a lot of visuals, you'll need cameras, tablets, illustrator programs, and editing software to bring your ideas to life.

Every job requires a variety of resources, and you'll need to make sure those are available to you, especially if you're going to be mobile. If your plan is to work from your home, storage is not as much of an issue. But when you're working from the road, space is a huge consideration. Will being on the road hinder your workflow? Will it limit what you can do because you don't have space for the equipment? Now is the time to think critically about the logistics and what is actually feasible for you.

Finally, you need to be brutally honest with yourself about income. I wish I could tell you that all freelancers are filthy rich, and that we just keep working because we're dedicated to our craft. I'm sure there are a few who are, but I have yet to hear a "getting started in freelancing" story that doesn't sound like the typical "young actor moving to the city" tale.

When you first appear on the scene, you can be Nobel Prize level talented, but you'll still need to network. You'll need to create a name for yourself. That means taking on the little tiny jobs that will prove that you actually have a scrap of talent. Over time, these clients will (hopefully) ask you to take on projects that are slightly larger in scope, and you'll get more credit, more money, and earn a better reputation.

Ask any small business owner from your list of contacts in Section Two. The first few years are going to be rough as you establish yourself. Working with a contracting site like Fiverr or Upwork can potentially speed up this process, but there will be stipulations and contracting fees involved.

You may land a glorious gig right off the bat, but that doesn't mean the work will always be there. My third contract was a long-term, high budget project for a real estate firm. It was a beautiful experience, but the contract eventually ended. That's simply the reality of freelance work- it is not a permanent position, and you will have to constantly hustle to find new gigs.

Can you afford this lifestyle? Will you be comfortable without the certainty of a paycheck? Are you pretty good with saving money for a rainy day? If your ideal scenario is to only work when you have to, then freelancing is perfect for you. But if you need to have a $2000 paycheck every other Friday in order to feel comfortable, then you may want to re-examine this option.

Hand-in-hand with pay come the other parts of compensation, such as benefits, taxes, and time off. These are very real parts of the working experience, at least in the United States, and you won't be exempt from needing medical and dental care or from paying taxes just because you're sitting in a van or skoolie. Research what options are available to you before you make the plunge, and get a feel for the tax requirements before you find yourself in a bind. There are plenty of materials out there to help freelancers find their feet, some of which I've included in the "Resources" section at the end of this book.

Freelancing can be incredibly rewarding, and the whole "free" part of it makes it ideal for folks who aren't made to work in a traditional office setting. Plus, technology has advanced to the point that it is now easier than ever to connect with others who are looking for your specific set of skills and talents.

Just remember, nothing comes truly for free. You will have to hustle. You will have to put yourself out there. The work is hard, and oftentimes you'll look back at your corporate paycheck with nostalgia and longing. But if that control factor is truly at the heart and soul of your decision to take your work on the run, freelancing is a great fit!

## Chapter Three: A Side-Hustle You Can Do All Day- or Not!

Side-hustles are the latest phenomenon amongst the working population, and it's easy to see why. These are the fun-sized versions of jobs, so to speak. Not only do you get to choose a money-making process that is fun and enjoyable for you, but you can work as much or as little as you want.

You can turn nearly any type of task into a side hustle, depending on your skills and interests. If you're a crafty or creative type, those talents can translate into a side-hustle very easily. As an example, one friend of mine is a very talented seamstress, and she has made an impressive living for herself doing basic mending and repairs as she and her husband travel in their big rig RV from campsite to campsite throughout the year. Another friend charges $5 per animal to walk dogs and keep pets entertained from her massive skoolie.

Coming up with a side-hustle may require a bit of creativity on your part, but everyone has a marketable skill. Side-hustles aren't necessarily tied to van life, either, anyone with the desire to can do them.

To come up with your side hustle, you need to look deep into your passions, and find a talent you enjoy that's profitable. I wrote an entire book about this process, called "How to Choose the Ultimate Side-Hustle: Making Money and Being Your Own Boss," but I'll lay out the groundwork here so you can decide if this is an option you'd like to pursue.

Similar to freelancing, there are nearly infinite opportunities that make ideal side-hustles. Here are just a few different niches and options that you might consider:

| Type of Hustle | Examples |
| --- | --- |
| Creative | home made arts and crafts, such as knitting or needlework, woodworking, painting or drawing, ceramics, jewelry making, quilting, soap making or creating bath goods, teaching crafting/creative classes. |
| Resale | rehab/refurbish of furniture, clothing, collectibles, vintage ware |
| In-person | pet sitting, housecleaning, babysitting, tutoring, pet grooming, car washing, yard work, drive for Uber/Lyft or a food delivery service, mystery shopping |
| Online help | tutoring, resume writing, affiliate marketing, email marketing, virtual assistant, blogging, drop shipping |

Some of these are going to work best if you plan on working from a stationary location, but you might be surprised at what you can take on the road. I know a woman who makes a small fortune in resale, and she's been living the van life for ten years. In fact, she attributes her success to her ability to travel anywhere, because she can accumulate collectibles and trinkets all over the country, knock the dirt off of them, and sell them via her website. She has her methods of storing them, taking good photographs, and then it's just a matter of keeping track of stock and shipping them as they sell.

Taking a side-hustle on the road does have a special set of considerations, as this example shows. She needs to make sure nothing is damaged so that she can sell the items and make money. That may seem impossible when you're on the road, since vans aren't usually climate controlled, and are generally in motion, jostling down bumpy roads. She has a system involving a padded drawer, towels, and plenty of bubble wrap. While you may not want to take on huge furniture restoration projects on the road, you might have a great time turning t-shirts into teddy bears. Let your mind wander a bit and see how creative you can truly be.

Having an in-person side-hustle while living on the road is another place where you might get stuck in the logical considerations, but it's not impossible. All across the country, you can find huge campgrounds where many part-time wanderers make their seasonal homes. These parks are filled with families, children, and pets. A babysitter or tutor would take a lot of stress off of parents' minds if they'd like to have some alone time. Watching their dogs will leave them free to explore places where Fido might not be welcome. And what harried mother wouldn't enjoy having someone else deep-clean their camper while they enjoy a few moments of peace and quiet? Even if you're just parked for a few nights, making your services known can bring in some spare cash quickly.

Online side-hustles are one place where road warriors can truly shine... as long as they have access to a good Wi-Fi connection! While people have been using the internet to make money since the early days of Angelfire, many of the options mentioned in the previous table are fairly new types of online gigs. Tutoring and resume writing are pretty familiar opportunities, but now there is newer video conference technology, like Zoom and Skype, that have changed how online courses and tutoring sessions are conducted. A virtual assistant gig is very much similar to that of a personal assistant- only with all communication taking place over text, chat, teleconferencing software, or email.

Affiliate and email marketing, as well as drop-shipping and blogging are definitely some examples of phenomena that have only appeared in recent internet history. Though each of these can be a side-hustle of its own, many people combine a little bit of each craft to create their own brand.

Affiliate marketers are hired by larger, online-based companies to essentially do their marketing for them. Rather than hiring professional ad departments and high price-tag marketing gurus (or sometimes in addition to), these companies hire regular everyday folks to come up with an ad campaign. That means you'll choose ad space, banners, and find interesting ways to capture the attention of the public, on behalf of the larger company. In exchange, they'll give you a personal marketer code, so that when anyone clicks on your ad to purchase their products, you will get a commission from the sale. Some of these affiliate marketing opportunities can be incredibly lucrative, especially when high-ticket items like cars, boats, or vacations are at stake!

Email marketing combines a bit of copywriting, a bit of marketing, and a bit of tech know-how. If you've purchased anything online, you've probably gotten at least one or two email follow-ups from that particular vendor. Email marketing is incredibly popular and effective, with sales and special offers coming to our inboxes all the time. In this gig, you'll be tasked with coming up with attractive copy and procuring a list of dedicated subscribers, which is usually provided to you. You then make sure the communications go out regularly, do any cleanup of unsubscribers or failed email addresses, and review the open rates and effectiveness of your campaigns. You may be asked to try different marketing approaches to increase appeal, and in some cases, tasked with responding to inbound email.

Drop-shipping is a very interesting approach to having your own online retail store, and an option that I'm seeing more and more frequently as a side hustle both in and out of the van community. In this model, you set up an online store- a website where you sell... stuff. Anything you can think of. You market your goods, attract customers and so on. But when people buy your "stuff," it's actually coming from a third party supplier- usually the manufacturer. You don't have to make anything, nor do you have to ship anything. All you have to do is set up the website, bring in the customers, and make sure they're happy.

And last- but certainly not least- there's blogging. This concept isn't new, but the idea that you can get paid for musing at length about a specific topic is still somewhat of an innovation. Bloggers get paid through selling ad space on their blogs, finding sponsors, and quite often with a touch of affiliate marketing.

There is a very blurry line—if any at all these days—between "social media influencers" and "bloggers." You can test this phenomenon by looking up a recipe. Any recipe will do! You'll likely find someone's food blog, where they'll meander through a touching story, followed by their experiences preparing this dish, complete with pictures and step-by-step detailed instructions. As you read, you'll notice that they mention very specific brands for some ingredients. That's the ticket to getting paid.

As a van lifer, you have a very particular niche at your fingertips when it comes to blogging and/or social media influencer potential. Our lifestyle is pretty unique, and setting up social media accounts, blogs, and websites is a typical practice in our community. Not only is it a great way to keep in touch with our friends and family back home and around the world, but it's the easiest way to save memories and photos of our journeys. I would be lying if I said I didn't occasionally have to peek at Brad's journal or my own blog to remember a certain location where we camped, or to double-check a particular hike to make sure I correctly recalled the spot.

There are ways to monetize your van life blog or social media account, such as checking in with potential sponsors and running some ads. You might also have a devoted group of followers who would love to purchase merchandise with your van name, blog handle, or logo printed on it!

To be perfectly clear, you do not have to be a van lifer to run a successful blog or social media account. There are plenty of lifestyle topics that are interesting and read well on blogs. You can even write a blog about how you transitioned from working in an office to working at home!

When it comes to choosing a side-hustle, innovation and strategy are key. It is rare to find success overnight. In fact, you'll likely have to work harder at finding followers, customers, and clients than you would as a freelancer. That being said, nearly everyone loves their side-hustle and wouldn't trade it for the world, though it's very simple to step away from a side-hustle when it no longer serves you!

## Chapter Four: Here, There, and Everywhere

You've probably seen an older television show or movie, in which a character proclaims to be "just traveling through" and "looking for some odd jobs" while they're in town. Like me, you might have thought that this was some old-fashioned ideal from days when the nomadic lifestyle was relatively popular, with folks riding the rails or even a horse out West to see what they could rustle up. In reality, this is still common amongst van lifers and explorers!

When it comes to living in a van, skoolie, RV, or any type of home on wheels, most people find themselves feeling a little disoriented by constantly moving. They'll find a spot to park for awhile, so they can get their bearings, along with a nice, hot shower and some clean laundry. Brad and I have done this many times- sometimes not on purpose, such as when the van has required extensive repairs. It provides a nice change of pace when you get to know a town or area a little bit before moving on.

Some people park cyclically in order to make a quick living before moving on. They'll find a reasonable location to park or camp, or even take up a bed in a hostel for a bit. Then, they'll find a temporary job for a month or even a few months, earning a regular paycheck and saving as much money as possible. After some time, with their financial stores replenished, they'll hit the road again.

There are quite a few jobs that lend themselves well to this lifestyle, such as seasonal warehouse and industrial work. Many temporary placement agencies are thrilled to have a reliable worker on hand for a short period of time. There's no pressure on anyone to find a long-term assignment, which can be beneficial for an employer who just needs someone to fill in while another person is on leave, or during peak season.

All of these types of positions will provide training, but some require a specific skill set that can make you a valuable asset as you seek out these temporary shifts. For example, warehouse or industrial jobs might require someone who is certified to drive a forklift or operate specialized equipment. Not everyone has those skills on their resume, so you'll be an instant hire if you show up in a new town with these types of qualifications.

Depending on how long you feel comfortable staying in one spot, these types of contracts can be very rewarding, both monetarily and through the contacts and experience you'll gain. I have a few young male friends who pop up at various warehouses across the country. They love how picking, stocking, and machine operating all day for a few months can keep them in peak shape, while padding their bank accounts for their next big adventure.

There are a few things to keep in mind when looking into these options, however. First, most temporary positions will require you to sign a contract for a specific period of time. While many states are "at will" employers, meaning you or the employer may terminate your contract for any reason and without warning, these contracts will make you stay put for a while. If you're not comfortable with looking at the same streets for more than a few days, this might not be the right fit for you.

Then there's the exact opposite issue: you might get attached. I had the opportunity to watch this play out with one of my college buddies. He bought the van and traveled. He stopped in a town in New Mexico to do some odd jobs. He met a very nice young lady. He and his wife are now permanent residents of a town in New Mexico.

On the other hand, I have several friends who have made the conscientious decision to not get attached. They prefer to be as brief as possible in order to avoid a mishap in which they find themselves permanently settled in a single location, at least for the time being. This is a perfectly valid narrative as well, so long as you are fully aware of what type of personal situation you want to maintain.

Lastly, it's very important to be clear to your employers that you are not in this for the long haul. You want to set up the expectation that you will be on hand as long as the contract allows, and then you will be gone. If you've got a terrific work ethic and knock it out of the park on all of your duties, the employer may try to coax you to stay longer, but that choice is entirely yours. You don't want to give anyone false hope that you're going to stick around, or pin you for a promotion when there are long-timers who may also deserve those opportunities.

## Chapter Five: Something for Everyone

As you can see, there's a little bit of everything available to those who work from home, on the road, or anywhere in between. Yes, adapting a specific job to your preferred remote situation may require a little finesse and creativity. There will be some research involved, some planning, and some strategy to get all of the moving pieces to fit just right.

Now that you've reviewed some options and examples of careers that can be taken anywhere, and professionals who make their jobs, work wherever they go, the brainstorming exercises from the first section might be making a little more sense. In order to be successful while doing your work on the run or even from your home office, you need to be thoroughly grounded in reality while constantly having your creative brain on in case you need to troubleshoot or find a solution to a problem you've never had before.

Even if nothing about your job changes at all, the situation is going to be very different. The problems will be new, and even solutions to familiar challenges will require a different outlook. But, if you're mentally prepared for what lies ahead, adapting to change and overcoming obstacles while still being productive will be the ultimate version of success!

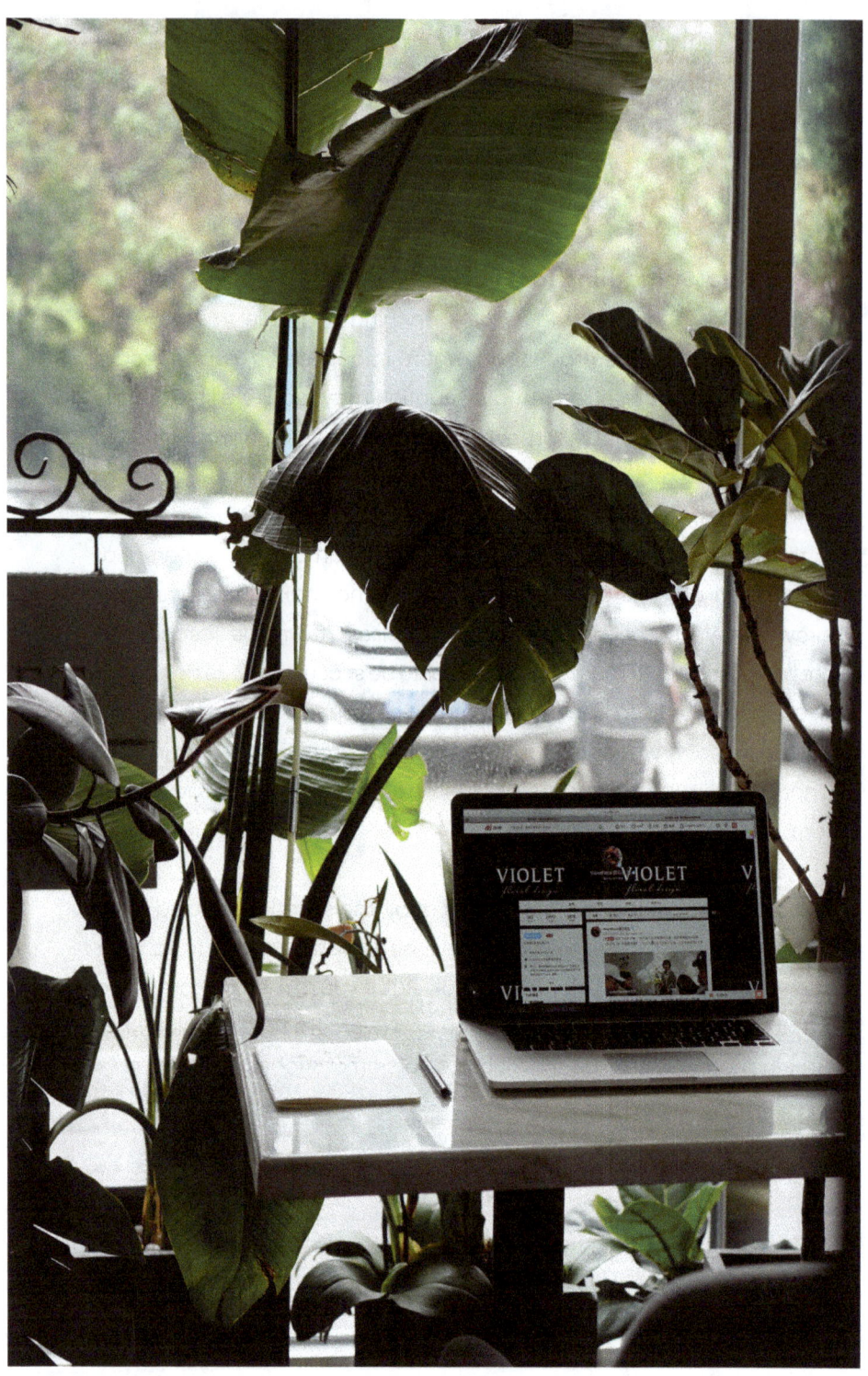

# Section Four: Setting the Stage

At this point, you're probably done with hard decisions, emotional introspectives, and difficult conversations. I am happy to report that, for the most part, that particular inner turmoil is behind you. That doesn't mean every day will be fantastic, and that your job will be nothing but fun and productive. Instead, you are now equipped with a significant amount of information and a new understanding about yourself. Now it's time to do some prep work that requires less soul searching and more construction.

Now that you have been granted the opportunity to take your career out of the office- or made the tough decision to drop everything and start anew- you need to prepare for that actual transition. You've done the tough work in getting mentally organized for this change, so now let's get physically prepared!

## Chapter One: Creating Your Work Space

Regardless of the job you plan to do, or whether you're planning on working from your home, a van, a skoolie, or a yurt, you're going to need to figure out the logistics of your work space.

At the bare minimum, you're going to need to find a spot where you can comfortably spread out all of your equipment and work materials, with adequate access to all of the resources you need to get you through your day. You may be thinking, "well, I did see that really cool desk at that antique store, so I think I'll get that." That's fine. Bookmark that. But before you start filling up your space with the things that inspire you, you have to *find* that space.

If you're planning on taking your job back to your home, you might think this is a super-easy decision. You'll turn the corner of the spare room into an office, or prop up a collapsible desk in front of the sofa, or maybe you'll just set up shop at the dining room table. Logically, all of these are fine ideas, depending on your available space. But will you actually want to work there?

When Brad first started working from home, he set up his office in an upstairs room we used for workout equipment. He chose this spot for several reasons:
- It was quiet and away from the rest of the flow of the house
- He could have his own room AND his own bathroom
- He could shut the door to keep out our dog (who loved to bark when anyone was on speakerphone)
- When he worked late, it didn't disrupt the things I needed to do

Logically sound, right? In fact, on paper, it couldn't be more ideal. Unfortunately, the reality was completely different.

It turns out that the top floor of the house didn't get the same amount of air circulation as the rest of the house. While the windows were situated at the east and west ends of the room, and let in a great deal of breeze, they also let in the sun all day long, baking Brad from sunrise to sunset. The ceiling of the room was also too low to install a fan, so the only option at the time was to run noisy floor fans that had to be turned off for conference calls and Skype meetings.

Adding to the noise was the fact that the windows looked directly over the street, so any ambient neighborhood sounds immediately made their way onto conference calls. That included our beagle scratching at the closed door any time he felt he should be included on those calls. What was an ideal space for our workout equipment was a terrible place to try to concentrate for 8-12 hours straight. It didn't take long for Brad to discover that working at the kitchen table was a far better option for him, though he did briefly experiment with our semi-finished basement and even the garage.

Working in the van, on the other hand, is an entirely different matter. Brad has a tote that he calls his "office." It includes a folding stool, his laptop case, all of his charging cords, a canopy that can be easily unfolded and set up, and a cushion for the stool. His "desk" is a foldable unit that's reminiscent of a card table and those metal tv trays my grandparents used to occasionally eat dinner in the living room.

Each day- weather willing- he sets up his "office" under the canopy, taking care to remain within the range of our WiFi signal. If the weather is poor, he either sets up his laptop on top of our storage units and works inside the van, or he'll head to town to find a location with free Wi-Fi until the weather breaks. One such location that is surprisingly perfect is the laundromat. He can take advantage of WiFi to work while simultaneously plowing through our endless stream of dirty laundry.

Then there are people like me. I work best when I change location several times throughout the day. I tend to lock into one spot, pound out a few thousand words, take a stretch break, find a spot that appeals to me more, then head to that spot for another few thousand words. While Brad thinks a stool is comfortable, my achy back and I disagree. I'll usually start out in the bed area of the van with an assortment of pillows. Then, as the inside of the van heats up under the sun, I'll take my folding chair and lap desk out to catch the breeze. If the weather isn't great, and we're not set up at the laundromat (or a cafe, restaurant, or on a few notable occasions, a brewery), I'm the type that will find every potential working position in that tiny space.

The idea of having a fixed office space makes me feel incredibly trapped and slightly claustrophobic, which you might find funny, considering I live in a van. But let's look at the difference between our jobs. Brad does a ton of objective problem solving. He needs quiet and concentration and the ability to focus on really big problems. On the completely opposite side of the career map, I'm creative. I need to keep myself inspired and focused. If I stare at the same thing too long, I get bored. When I get bored, my mind starts wandering. When my mind starts wandering, so do I, and pretty soon I'm chasing butterflies or Googling information none of my current clients care about, like the type of car Columbo drove, or the lyrics to a song I listened to in high school.

I share these examples to demonstrate that work space is not one-size-fits-all, and that you may have to try a few different things out before you find the area that works best for you. You may have additional variables in your equation, like pets or children who are bound to make noise and require attention. If you have a bad back, or history of carpal tunnel flare ups, ergonomics are definitely something to keep in mind, as well. Don't settle for just any spot because you like the view. Make sure it works from a 360-degree approach!

Therefore, my recommendation to you is to come up with a few options for your work space. As mentioned earlier, the only real requirement is that you have enough room to set up all of your equipment and have access to any connectivity that is required of your job.

Let's look at what you need to work, equipment-wise. For nearly everyone, that's going to include a laptop. Even if you plan on pursuing a creative side-hustle, you'll still need a way to market your product. You might also require a label printer to print off addresses and postage for shipping. You'll also need whatever supplies are required to make your amazing product, and a way to store those supplies, whether at home or on the road.

I recommend starting with a list of everything you need to get things moving. For me, that looks like this:

- Laptop
- Charging cord
- Cell phone
- Caffeinated beverage
- Headphones
- Pillow to prop up laptop on my actual lap
- Notebook with dividers and pen

As you can see, I've included everything I can think of that I'll need. This prevents me from doing the whole "Ooh. I need to go get..." distraction routine. If I have my set up all planned out, I am entirely ready to go for the day.

Once you've gathered everything you need, figure out how to make it fit. If you're a desk person, this is probably super easy. If you're working from home, it may take a little finessing. But if you're working on the road, you've got to figure out where to put your drink so it won't spill on something important, and the phone has to go somewhere it can't fall in between cracks or make its way under something. The charge cords have to reach the power center, and don't you dare wander too far away from the WiFi!

Before your first day of working away from the office, walk through this process. Figure out what works and what doesn't. I will say that the greatest detractor from productivity in a work from home scenario is finding your stuff. Even at home, Brad would set his phone down when getting a cup of coffee and then spend the next fifteen minutes searching for it. Factor in the small nooks and crannies of a van or skoolie, and you can understand why preparedness and organization are key!

While you're in the process of conducting this dry run or walk through, make it a point to actually boot up your equipment. Make sure you can actually connect to any services you need to connect to, such as WiFi or a phone signal. At our house in Ohio, it was impossible to get a consistent phone signal in the basement or the front bedroom, and the WiFi didn't work directly in front of the fireplace. If you haven't explored the possibilities, you may not be aware of these types of dead zones until you're on the clock, so take the time to check things out before you try to log on for your first official day.

Setting up your work space may be one of the most objectively simple tasks on your list, but that doesn't mean it will be effortless. Giving your work space some conscious thought and deliberate design will aid your daily productivity. You'll not only stay on track by having everything where it needs to be, but you won't be distracted by trying to make things "perfect" when something doesn't feel or work right. You know your workflow better than anyone, so make sure your space is adequate for getting the job done.

## Chapter Two: Understanding How to Work in a New Place

How do you work? If you've worked in a separate location your entire career, you may say, "well, I go to my place of employment, I clock in, and I start working." And that's a great start! But that's all about to change.

Walk yourself through a typical day in the office. You walk in, sure. Do you go straight to your desk, or do you detour to get a coffee or maybe some breakfast on your way? Once you arrive at your desk or work station, what's the first thing you do? Do you take a few moments to get yourself organized for the day, or do you jump right in by checking email or voicemail while you're still taking off your jacket?

Whether we like it or not, humans are most productive when they adhere to a routine. That's not necessarily a hard-and-fast rule, but once you start to examine your current work patterns a bit more, you'll realize that you tend to do things similarly each day.

For example, I wake up, start the coffee, wash up, and do a little brisk walk/jog around our camping area to get the blood flowing. Then I open up my laptop and start getting things organized while I desperately chug my coffee, waiting for its eye-opening effects to kick in. Brad wakes up, grabs a cup of coffee in a to-go mug, and wanders around for a good half hour, stimulating his senses into waking up with a nice walk. He washes up on his way back to the van, then sets up his office, and dives right in. One of our van life friends has the most astounding pre-work ritual I've ever heard of. He hikes at least 5 miles, chugs a can of craft beer, makes breakfast, and is ready to go by 9am EST every single day. He owns his own marketing firm, and despite his odd routine, does quite well for himself.

On your first day working remotely, you may feel a bit lost and stranded, especially if you've never worked outside of the traditional office setting. You might feel equal parts anxious to get the day started and excited by the idea that you can sleep in a little bit, since you don't have to get dressed up or drive anywhere. You may have added some new duties, like getting the kids ready for school, walking the dog, or getting breakfast ready for your household.

Regardless, this is another part of the day where a quick run-through before this becomes your actual process is beneficial. You don't have to practice until you have it down perfectly, but for many of us, learning through experience can help us develop our stride.

Once you've considered the start to your day, the rest of the work day should unfold somewhat naturally... or will it? If you're the type of person who does very well working on your own, who can moderate mental breaks, distractions, and productivity without interacting with others, then yes, you should be as good as gold.

On the other hand, if you're the type of person who likes to visit with other coworkers, and often collaborates on projects with other people in your office, you might suddenly feel incredibly lonely. You won't have the opportunity to stand up and walk to someone else's desk to ask their opinion on a specific issue. Depending on the technology available, you can send them an instant message, email, or call them, but it's not going to be the same.

You may discover that your new work environment is oppressively quiet. If you're completely alone, you may feel a brand new sense of isolation and almost abandonment. The people who once shared almost all of your waking hours are now spending that time without you, while you are all alone. They're laughing and joking at impromptu breakroom meetings, going to lunch together, bringing in treats to share with the office, and you aren't taking part in any of that.

If you are a very collaborative, team-oriented type of person, you will find this newfound solitary environment more distracting than anything you could have possibly imagined. Your dog could actually begin singing- not just the songs of his people, but Ave Maria- and it wouldn't be nearly as confounding as this isolation.

Then again, you may be the type of person who enjoys micromanagement, and you feel most in control and confident when someone is dictating exactly what you should be doing at every given moment. Many people feel like a boat floating away from its mooring when they first start working remotely. If you're going from a very tight-knit environment with clear, constant direction to freelancing, you're going to feel a bit lost at first. Now, if you feel that you have "escaped" that type of scenario, where you found the expectations of coworkers and management unrealistic and oppressive, then you're in the right spot. But if you're the type who second-guesses yourself every time you hit the spacebar on your keyboard, the transition will seem strange.

One recommendation I have for those who are more collaborative, or require more direction, is to try very hard to maintain that same level of connection. That can mean setting up quick phone calls with people to check in, or having day-end meetings with your boss to check up on everything. You might even suggest a weekly video conference with your team so you can all touch base on what you've done for your respective projects.

If you're changing fields entirely, don't let that be a reason to give up your professional connections. Remember that list of contacts you made earlier? Touch base with them. Be honest with them, too. "I'm feeling a little lost about starting this 'running my own business' thing. Can we take some time to talk about your experiences when you first started running your own show?" Anyone who has made this type of transition will relate to the myriad of feelings you're having, ranging from freedom to fear and independence to isolation. You're not nearly as alone as you feel.

Not only is your work style going to change significantly, but your work environment, as well. Every office building has some level of ambient noise, due to various parties being on the phone, holding meetings, etc. All of the elevator dings, street noise, mechanical whirrs, and the hum of the HVAC become subtly embedded in your brain, and you learn to work in that type of environment.

So when you've been working for a few hours, and you don't hear the elevator or hear your children's morning cartoon instead of a dull murmur of productivity, you may feel a bit displaced.

Try experimenting with different ambient sounds. I mentioned earlier that I prefer binaural beats, because music with words distracts me. Brad prefers 1980s hair bands, because the beat is fast and furious. I wrote an entire textbook to "Star Trek: The Next Generation," because I wanted to emulate the tone of Captain Jean-Luc Picard. You have complete permission to create the brain space you need to work efficiently.

One particular peril of working on the run is that you don't really have control over your environment. Brad and I were thrilled to find that we had a campsite in Alabama all to ourselves (hooray for the off-season!), until the maintenance crew came in at 11am on the dot to start mowing, trimming branches, and making all kinds of ruckus. Some campsites are filled with children and dogs who will make lots of noise starting at exactly 7am every day... in fact, some of those children and dogs may be your own! You can't control what the people around you are doing, so this is a situation where you'll have to evaluate if you need to take things to town, or if you can work with the windows up and headphones on for a bit.

Learning how to work in an entirely different environment can present some unexpected challenges. We'll look into dealing with some of the emotional and psychological changes in the next section, as well. In the process of creating your physical work space, you can take charge of as many challenges as you can recognize before getting started. That includes finding the ideal desk/chair/room situation, figuring out your start of day flow, and understanding what type of worker you are so you can meet any distractions head-on.

## Chapter Three: Time to Work!

The next challenge is creating your work schedule. This is particularly important for freelancers, side-hustlers, and van folks of all industries.

The temptation to slack off will be incredibly strong at first. The distractions will be off the charts. For those starting out with freelancing and side-hustle gigs, when clients and projects are at an all-time low, you may feel that this is the opportunity to do nothing. Granted, folks in this position do have a bit more freedom than others, but doing nothing all day, everyday isn't the best option.

Instead, everyone who is making this full-on transition needs to think about creating a schedule. This schedule must not only make sense with your lifestyle, but with the tasks you need to complete, too.

This whole process started with an awareness of changes you need to make in your lifestyle in order to truly live. Whether that means carving out time for appointments, working fewer hours, working in the middle of the night, or taking a great big break in the middle of the day, your schedule should reflect exactly what your mind and body need in order to survive and thrive. You should have time to eat, take care of your personal needs, and get a satisfactory amount of work completed each day.

You also need time to rest. That amount differs for all of us. Some people are mentally and physically equipped to go for days on end, then crash for a day, get up, and do it all over again. Others may need a cat nap during the day to recharge. Whatever your body needs, allow it. While taking a thirty minute snooze at your desk during lunch break might be frowned upon, getting thirty minutes of shut eye on your sofa after eating a sandwich is no big deal. No one will ever know! You have the control factor. You have the freedom. Do whatever it takes to help yourself flourish in this new situation.

Then there are the tasks you need to complete. The "work" part of every "work/life" balance must not be ignored. Starting a career in freelancing or performing a side-hustle is not unlike the experience of a freshman starting college. You get your assignment and the due date, but how you get there is up to you. You could study up on the topic rigorously, attending every possible lecture, taking copious notes, and adding a bit to your project each day. Or, you can devote that energy and ambition to whatever feels like fun, and cap it all off with a series of all-nighters right before the big due date.

In this metaphor, of course, there are no lectures to attend, but the concepts are pretty similar. If a client gives you a due date that's a month out, you can choose to start research and preparations now, or you can wait until the last minute. Maybe you work best under pressure and have chosen only projects that you can complete quickly. As long as you get that final project in on time, and the client loves it, you'll pass the metaphorical class.

There are plenty of exercises you can try out to help keep your head in the game. In speaking with others who have made the transition to working from home or on the road, I learned that sometimes you have to trick yourself into being more disciplined than you want to be. Here are some of the tricks I've compiled from my own experiences and conversations with others who have left the office behind:

1. **Give yourself tighter deadlines.** Even if the assignment isn't due for a week, get it done faster. That way, you don't have the ability to slack off and hate yourself for it.

2. **Make your breaks meaningful.** Absolutely get up and stretch and move every 30-60 minutes- but don't take this as an opportunity to find a new distraction. Don't turn on the TV, don't even think about logging on to social media, and definitely don't get yourself caught up in a personal project that's going to drag your mind away for hours. Take a brief, brisk walk. Have a snack. Doodle. Meditate. Do some yoga. Do anything that you can immediately drop after 10-15 minutes without effort.

3. **Plan out a rough schedule for your week.** I personally hate lists and schedules, because when things go sideways, I become a giant ball of anxiety and guilt. However, if you create even the most bare-bones outline of your day or week, it will help you know what you need to accomplish. You'll also be abundantly aware of deadlines that are creeping up on you.

4. **Stick to your schedule.** This is INCREDIBLY hard for freelancers and side-hustlers, because you may have a few days where you are not required to get up early and pound out a project. You want to sleep in, breathe deep, and just stare at the wall. That's completely valid, but once work picks up again, you'll feel bitter that you don't have the same amount of slack off time you had earlier. Give yourself time to rest and recover- especially after difficult projects- but keep your mind involved and active.

5. **Choose a hobby that has nothing to do with your occupation.** Since I've made reading and writing my job, I don't find sitting down with a good book as relaxing as it used to be. Instead, I fire up an audio book and listen to a fabulous tale while I draw or color. After a long day of looking at a computer screen, I absolutely adore setting up my yoga mat outside and following along with an online yoga flow. Brad is a runner, so the unspoken rule is that he will hang up the phone, close his laptop, deconstruct his office, lace up his shoes, and come back after a few miles of jogging it out. You need something to look forward to and a method that truly helps you re-engage with the life part of the work-life balance.

These are just a few tips from those of us who have been there and done that. You may accidentally discover a technique that really works for you. Enjoy the control you have earned by leaving the office environment, and do what makes you feel more productive and encourages you to keep working. Inspiration is literally everywhere. If the "Hang In There, Baby" poster from your desk space did something for you, hang it up in your workspace. Make it your laptop wallpaper. You no longer have coworkers to get irritated by it, so go ahead and click your pen endlessly for 45 minutes. Keep your brain focused in a way that's meaningful for you, and the productivity will follow!

Creating the perfect physical, mental, and emotional space for success in your new endeavor requires a little more effort than you might initially imagine. You may need to spend the first few months of your new work scenario figuring out exactly what works for you, and ironing out all the details. This may be frustrating, but ultimately, you will find your stride. Oftentimes, this happens quite organically, as you settle in with your new routine. Other times, you will have to experiment with ways to motivate yourself out of bed, and to coax yourself into sitting down and working, even when you really don't want to do a single thing. Personally, I would say it was about a year before I really felt like I was doing things "right" for me. You may need more or less time. Just know that no one has ever found this to be a quick and easy process, and you are truly never alone!

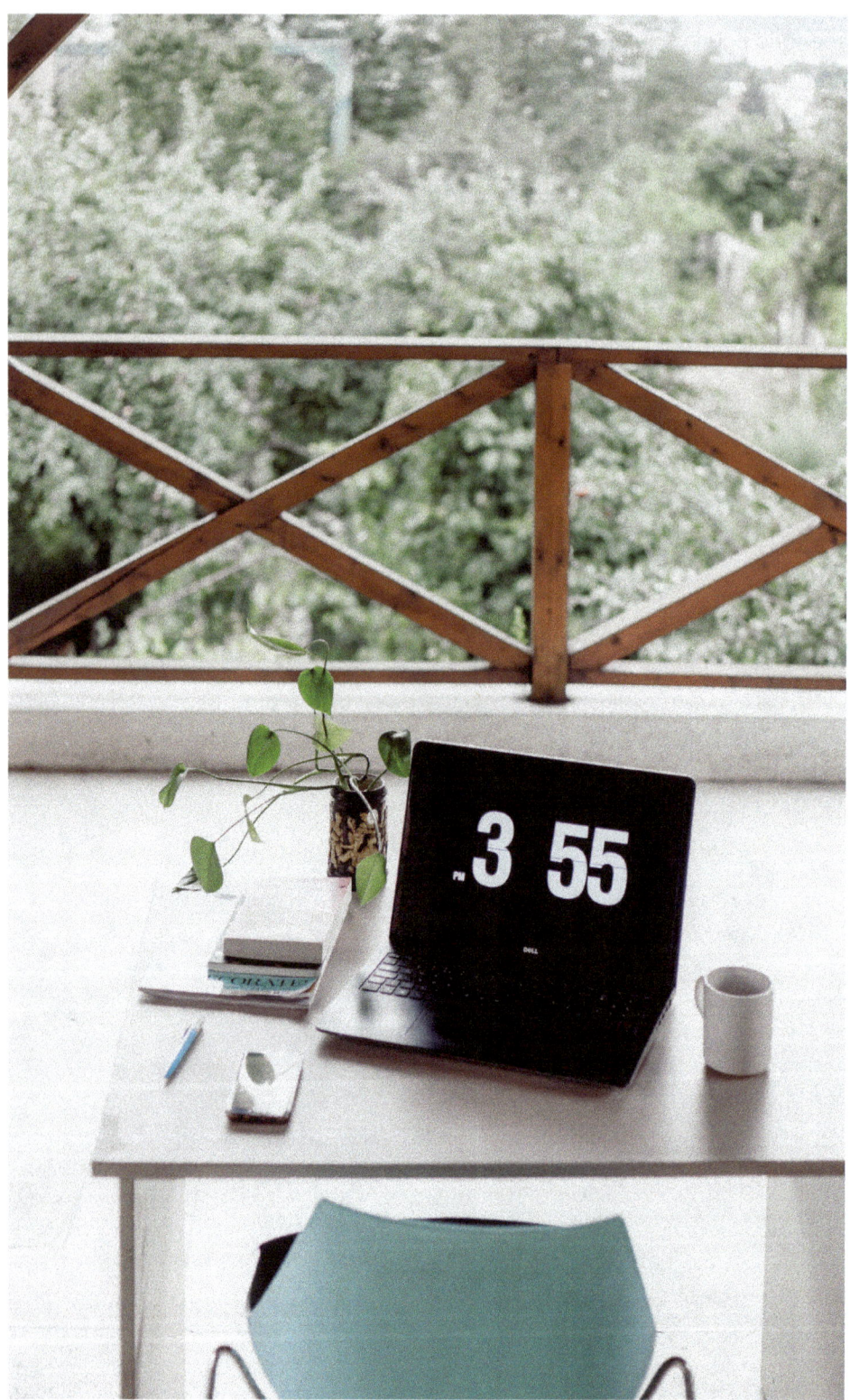

# Section Five: Finding Your Stride and Making It Work

Now that you've got your plan in hand, it's time to make it work. Don't be surprised if you experience some growing pains along the way, however. You've just changed your entire working model, so there are a few aspects of your overall attitude, daily experience, and long-term success that might change radically. Still, it is possible to turn these growing pains into incredible experiences, so that you might be truly successful in a career that rewards you not just financially, but emotionally, as well.

## Chapter One: The Social Aspect

Earlier, we touched on how your work environment will drastically change your interactions with others. Many of us thrive in an office environment due to the social aspect, either because of the opportunities for collaboration and direction, or through commiserating with our fellow employees. We make friends in the office, some of whom become very near and dear to us. The concept of an "office spouse" or "office bestie" is not unheard of, because many of us gain very close relationships with those who understand and appreciate exactly what we go through for the majority of our waking hours.

Once you take yourself out of that environment of closeness and camaraderie, you may feel a deep sense of isolation. This is perfectly natural. For those who are simply transitioning the same job they've had in the past to a home office, it's a great idea to continue to meet up with coworkers for lunch or happy hours, so that you can retain that social connection.

But what if you're changing jobs completely? If you're permanently leaving the office behind for a freelance lifestyle or the ultimate side-hustle, you may feel like you're saying goodbye. It's true that some things about your friendship will change. You won't be at the same level for venting sessions or office chatter, but you don't have to walk away from a beautiful bond just because the situation has changed. Meet up for coffee, connect via social media, and invite each other to social gatherings. You may be surprised to discover that your former coworkers will simply love seeing you at the occasional happy hour, and they'll have tons of questions about your new gig- along with a little residual jealousy.

Van life folks have it the hardest when it comes to the changes in the social aspect of working on the run. You are voluntarily stuck in a small, enclosed vehicle, all day, every day, with the same person. Granted, the opportunity for isolation exists, as demonstrated by Brad taking off with his office-in-a-tote while I occupy the van, but the only people you have to complain/vent/exalt to regularly are those who are also seated in the same vehicle.

At first, they'll be fascinated with your stories, especially if you are both new to this job or environment. You'll excitedly chatter over an evening meal, relishing that pre-bedtime glass of wine or mug of cocoa as you rehash the day to mentally process everything that has happened. Eventually, you will reach what I call the "Who Cares?" phase, in which one person speaks while anyone else present rapidly forgets how to listen. This stage can be difficult, because it's fairly easy to tell when no one is paying attention to you. Over time, this morphs into a sense of personal involvement, when you realize you've become deeply entrenched in each other's work, despite having only the faintest clue of what they're doing and how it happens. You may find yourself coming up with nicknames for people you've never met, and starting sentences with "you should tell them... ." It may not be healthy, but it's a very real step in the bonding process of people who work in solitude.

In the office, Brad was "kind of a big deal." He had people stopping at his desk from the moment he walked in the door until the automatic timers shut off the lights for the evening. He was invited to nearly every team's social functions, both work related and personal.

When he started working from home, a lot of that stopped. Not only did he lose the constant stream of visitors, but the invites started trailing off, as people who would extend those invitations in elevators, breakrooms, and the parking garage lost sight of him. Though he's not an extrovert by any means, losing the social aspect was pretty depressing. He felt an extreme sense of isolation. Thankfully, he adapted by the time he started working on the road, but it was a lengthy period of coping.

For me, the sense of loneliness hit almost immediately after we pulled out of the driveway. I'm also an introvert, but I rely heavily on my network for regular interaction and connection. I was used to seeing the same coworkers each day, laughing, complaining, crying, and sharing snacks with them. Being on the road took all of that away from me. In fact, I stopped having my 3pm snack altogether! While that was a great move for weight loss, the sense of losing my group was painful.

There are a few things you can do to ease this transition into solitude. A few of the methods we used include:

1. **Find your favorite noise.** I've mentioned music, podcasts, and audio books a few times. These are actually great ways to make your brain feel less lonely. You get to hear sounds and voices and get information, even when no one is around. One method I enjoy is putting a documentary on for background noise while I make meals. I love information. I love hearing other humans' voices. I can learn all about British castles while making dinner, and while the host will never hear my witty commentary, I get to hear his charming remarks.

2. **Stay connected.** Your network is key. Text your friends and family. Keep up with your social media. Heck, if the phone connection is strong enough, call them! One fun activity that helped get me through the first year of van travel was sending postcards to a friend. The messages started out short enough- after all, there's very little room on a postcard. Soon, I was explaining why the postcard made me think of her, and the story of how that postcard ended up in the mail to her. Plus, finding stamps and post boxes is a challenge in itself that can keep you occupied for hours (for extra fun, don't use a GPS)!

3. **Talk to strangers.** If reading that sentence makes you feel queasy and uneasy, you're not alone. The first few months of van living found me fully tongue tied. I felt uneasy speaking to anyone, because I was truly a "stranger in a strange land." I didn't know anyone, and I didn't belong. It wasn't until Brad ended up fielding a work call at a brewery in Montana that I suddenly felt a pressing need to make new friends. Perhaps the strong brew eased my apprehension, but soon I was chatting about van life with the woman sitting next to me, the bartender, and two little boys who came in with their father.

   Not everyone is receptive to meeting new people, and I'm certainly not saying you should put yourself on the threshold of danger. But being out and about, sharing a few friendly words with fellow hikers, folks at restaurants and cafes, neighbors at camping spots, and more can be soothing to the soul. It can also be highly productive, as your interaction may reveal some cool ideas for things to do, restaurants to try, and fantastic views. A chance interaction with a fellow in a restaurant in Idaho led to a quickly sketched map to a free camp spot in the National Forests. From there, Brad and I were treated to the most stunning sunset we have ever experienced. It can truly pay off to learn from the locals through casual conversation.

4. **Find events to attend.** From car rallies to county fairs, there is always something happening, somewhere. You can find inexpensive and free events to pop into briefly until your social craving is whetted. If you find that you're enjoying yourself, stay a spell. Brad and I have done all sorts of things that we wouldn't have done at home, from going to a rodeo, to attending a lecture on the socio-psychological turmoil experienced by those involved in the Western Expansion. We've appeared at art gallery events, beer releases, and even a book release for a tome about Sasquatch. If you need a crowd, it's easy to find one. Plus, these experiences become some of the highlights of your van life adventure.

I won't say it's easy to move forward, and I certainly can't say that this feeling of solitude will go away. Even if it's the thing that most excites you about van life during the planning stages, you'll have a certain feeling of disconnection as you physically distance yourself from the world you once knew. You don't have to give up your friendships, however. You just need to learn how to help them evolve.

## Chapter Two: The Growth Aspect

"Where do you see yourself in ten years?" Anyone who has been to a job interview, performance review, or motivational career event has heard that question. And despite the fact that we fumble through a few words about growth, success, and learning, the truth is, we often have no idea. Personally, I can't picture dinner when I wake up in the morning. How am I supposed to know what my life is going to look like in a decade? I don't know what the economy will look like, or what marketing trends will be, and I don't know if the van is going to last another ten years, and... there are a lot of "what ifs" on everyone's horizon.

One area in which you have control is your career. You have already demonstrated that when you made the decision to leave the traditional office setup. And while that's probably plenty to deal with for now, eventually you will want to progress somehow.

Whether you're maintaining your current role or planning on knitting scarves from the back of a van, your career is not immune to growth. Maybe you're small bananas now, but every job, craft, art, occupation, past-time, and opportunity has the ability to lead you somewhere on your life's path.

When I started freelancing, some of my first gigs were writing 300-word "About" pages for $5 a pop. They required about thirty minutes of research and ten minutes of writing. But I took as many as I could handle, and I wrote my heart out. Now I'm reading, editing, and writing books full time. Who knows where I'll be in a year, two years, or more?

Maybe you're happy knitting scarves in the back of your van. That is completely respectable. I love handmade items, and scarves are a great source of warmth for people who don't have central heat or think that ice hiking is fun. But maybe, as the slips and purls go by, you're thinking about how you can combine your knitting skills with your motivational skills, and create an opportunity in which your scarf sales can benefit others. Maybe you're planning a non-profit in which your scarves can be donated to the homeless, and create a mission from there. No job is small. No creation is without impact.

If growth is something you crave, I encourage you to pursue it. How? There are several ways:

- **Learn.** Distance learning is easier now than it ever has been, with online programs that can help you advance your knowledge in marketing yourself and your skills. If you find a weak spot that is preventing you from getting to where you dream of being, apply your energy towards learning more. Do the research. Take the courses. Listen to the lectures.
- **Network.** I've said it before: you are not alone. Find the community, and become part of the niche. Look for mentors and companions on this journey. If Frodo could convince Samwise to walk with him to Mordor, then surely you can find others who can get on board with your fantastic idea.
- **Stay connected.** Or rather, don't be oblivious. When I started writing, I had no idea that MLA-style was no longer a thing. All of the lessons I'd been taught, all of the terrible marks I'd received for grammatical errors were no longer valid. In this day and age, a lot of the rules have changed. For example, it's ok to start sentences with the word "However." If I had a time machine, I'd love to go back to college and apprise a few professors of these facts, but unfortunately, that technology doesn't exist. What this means is that when I started freelancing, I received a whole bunch of comments on my outdated style. That's entirely my fault- I didn't stay connected to learn about these changes. You'll have far better success with growth if you keep your finger on the pulse of your industry.

- **Be honest about it.** Tell your boss, your clients, and your network of your personal aspirations. You can't make your dreams a reality if you pretend they don't exist. If you explain to your boss that you'd like to make your way to Director level in the next three years, chances are very good that they'll be able to provide you with tips and goals that will take you down that path. If you're performing well for a client in a freelance scenario, and you mention that you're looking for something more, they may very well be happy to accommodate that growth with additional projects and increased responsibility.

But what if, in the lexicon of our youth, you "don't wanna?" You have control now. You don't have to grow. You don't have to aspire to take over a Fortune 500 company by the time you're fifty- unless you want to. You can write the Great American Novel, or you can cheerfully write web content and product descriptions for the rest of your working life. You can start a world-wide charity based on your scarf knitting, or you can do nothing more wild than finishing a sweater. It's all up to you.

In the office environment, I found that the need to rise up the proverbial ladder, to smash the glass ceiling and rule the world, and to continuously have motion within the corporate hierarchy was more of an expectation than my own personal desire. Sure, everyone loves an increase in pay, but the drastic increase in responsibilities that come with that bigger check sometimes outweighs the benefits.

When you first started to consider working remotely, as we did in the first chapter, you came to realize that the picture is a little bigger than your specific role within the org chart. This is especially true if your reasons for leaving the office are for family or personal issues. As that disconnect from the social aspect kicks in, you might start to feel like you'll never advance in your career, but that's simply not true. Compromising personal needs and your career should always work out in your favor.

A wise mentor of mine once told me, "for me, it's more important to become valuable for what I do, not how much of it I do." That is to say, prioritize your own well-being, enjoy your lifestyle, and don't burn out.

## Chapter Three: The Financial Aspect

Maybe I've read too many "how to" financial advice books (ironically, for a client), but one question that will always intrigue me is the value of a dollar.

We tend to think about the financial aspect of our career in terms of amounts. When given a task to perform for pay, we see dollar signs, coin heaps and bills paid instead of hours spent, emotions invested, and brain power taxed. Somehow, the promise of financial gain makes us forget that work is hard.

Also, we obviously need money to live. I'd love to write a book called "How to Quit Your Job and Have Fun Doing Whatever You Want," but that's not in the cards right now. While working from home will help you save the money you would have spent on commuting, work clothes, and treating yourself to lunch or coffee every day, there are always expenses to count on. We all need food and shelter. Some of us need to put gasoline in our shelters every few hundred miles!

What I'm asking you to consider through all of this is the balance you want to make between the effort you make and the payment you take. This is true for anyone with a paying job, but there tends to be this wild misconception that anyone who isn't in the office magically has more time than anyone else. You may feel pressured to take on more tasks to "prove" that you can work from a remote location and still be productive, or you may find people wordlessly assigning you more projects.

For freelancers and side-hustlers, this is also very true, especially in the first few years. The first few years are stressful not just because you're trying to establish yourself, but because your brain and your body are not trained for this sudden change. The gig you choose may require more physical activity, and it will definitely engage new areas of your brain.

Even though I was an English major in college, where reading, researching, and reporting massive quantities of facts and ideas was something I did multiple times a day, that part of my brain had only been moderately simmering while I was working in a corporate human resources environment. When I first began writing full time, I found myself absolutely exhausted to the point where my computer screen would turn to gibberish after a few hours. My brain was just over tired.

You will likely approach your freelancing gigs and side-hustle activities with a violent fervor at first, and that energy is absolutely wonderful. Just make sure that you aren't putting in more effort than you're being compensated for.

At the same time, you need to balance cost of living with your income. For those remaining in their stationary homes, you'll already be aware of your general living expenses. But keep in mind that working from home means you don't have to live within a reasonable commute to the office. Depending on whether you still have to (or wish to) make in-person appearances, you now have the ability to take control over that part of your life, too. Once that twice-a-day commute is taken out of the daily equation, many people feel they have the freedom to work from areas where the cost of living is not quite as steep as it may have been otherwise.

For those transitioning to van life, your expenses are going to be very different. How different, or in what ways, depends on what type of vehicle you have, what type of adventure you've planned, and many other factors that I covered in "How to Live the Dream: Things Every Van Lifer Needs to Know." Whether you choose the gig first or the van life first, you will need to eventually align your expenses and income.

This may require a bit of experimentation, especially if you are new to both van living and freelancing or your side-hustle. Don't become discouraged, even though it can be very tempting to just give up. You can always go back to the drawing board and reconsider your options. That's the beauty of working for yourself: you can "quit" one job and take up another with just a few clicks of the mouse and an ounce of resolution.

In fact, I found myself re-evaluating my life choices about every month the first year. I'm lucky, in that Brad's steady income was present, and we had purposefully saved for our van life for a few years before we hit the road. But if I came to the end of the month and realized that I was quickly burning out, then noticed that I'd only made $100 in the entire month, that meant I wasn't doing it right. There will always be months that are sparse, unless you have regular clients. You can choose to respond by picking up more clients or gigs, or adding something else to your repertoire. Alternately, you can find a home base and "sit out" for a while to give your brain the option to come up with another plan!

## Chapter Four: The Fear Aspect

One of the most common excuses that we tell ourselves is that "the time isn't right." This may seem especially resonant when you factor in the previously mentioned facts that you will be alone, that your career path may change, and that your financial situation will require a different level of attention than it has in the past.

When you start to have these sneaking feelings that maybe "the time isn't right," ask yourself if that's really the case, or if that's just the fear speaking. Both are extremely valid options, depending on your situation.

Let's look at a few ways that fear might be manifesting in your plans, and think of some questions to ask yourself to suss out whether it's real or anxiety:

| Your Brain Says | Is It Real? | Is It Fear? |
|---|---|---|
| "If you leave now, you'll be passed over for that promotion." | • Does your employer have a history of giving remote workers the cold shoulder?<br>• Do you have a history of shaky performance?<br>• Are you really fully invested in receiving that promotion? Is it one of your Top 5 Goals at this moment? | • What is the worst thing that will happen if you do not receive this promotion?<br>• Will receiving this promotion mean that you can't work from home or on the road?<br>• If you wait until you receive the promotion to change your work situation, what other details of your life will also be put on hold? |
| "Things are just really busy right now, and transitioning out of the office would disrupt everything." | • Would the majority of your current job duties be impossible to perform from another location?<br>• Is there no one else who can perform the tasks you regularly handle?<br>• Is the success of this particular project or period in the office currently weighing on your mind more than the lifestyle you wish to pursue? | • Are you the most important cog in this particular wheel?<br>• What would happen if a dire emergency kept you away from the office for an extended period of time? Would this task plunge into chaos?<br>• When this task is complete, will you be ready to leave the office behind? |
| "I've only been in this job for a year. What will it look like if I leave now?" | • Is this a career path that you intend to follow for a significant period of time?<br>• Is this particular job an incredibly valuable stepping stone to your overall life goals?<br>• Will staying in this job provide you with opportunities you can't get anywhere else? | • Are you intimidated by the idea of having a frank discussion about altering your job situation with your management team?<br>• Does the concept of failing at your attempt to work from the road or from home make you feel more uncomfortable than the idea of maintaining the status quo?<br>• What factors in the first exercise led you to believe that working remotely was the best decision in the first place? |

Ultimately, the question you need to ask yourself is, "Is it really better to wait?"

Sometimes, the answer is yes. You may not have the vehicle you need sitting in your driveway. You may have only $4 in your bank account until next Friday. You may have children who are attending school, family members who rely on you being exactly where you are now, or any of a variety of factors that make staying exactly where you are the right decision, right now.

That doesn't mean you can't start planning your exit strategy now. In fact, you have an advantage that many of us didn't necessarily consider when leaving the office behind. Nearly everyone has fantasized about walking into the boss's office on a particularly rough day, launching into a poignant rage-fueled (yet well-worded) speech about where anyone listening can put this job, grabbing the best chotchkies from their cubicle, and slamming the door behind them as they leave with a flourish.

You may be incredibly frustrated and confused and angry with the way things are going now. Or maybe you felt that way when you completed the exercises in Section One, but as you cool off, you realize there are a lot more moving parts than you originally considered. Maybe working remotely will eventually be the correct answer, but setting off at dawn tomorrow isn't the best option. That doesn't mean you have to officially close the book on this option. Instead, brainstorm the pieces that need to move- and where they need to go- so you can one day get to the job situation you crave.

I recommend anyone who is still wavering on whether the time is right take this short quiz:

1. Which is more important to you:
   a. Gaining wealth
   b. Earning higher status
   c. Living the best possible life

2. How far away is retirement for you? If you wait until then to pursue all of the things you're putting off by not working from home or the road, will you be:
    a. Perfectly happy
    b. Bitter and resentful
    c. Oh, I'm definitely not waiting that long. I'm a year out at max.

3. What is the number one thing that you need to make you feel comfortable with leaving the office?
    a. The moral support of friends, family, and coworkers
    b. Money
    c. A box to carry my stuff

4. Essay Question: What other changes have you put on hold because you're afraid?

There are no right or wrong answers to this quiz, of course. The intention is to get your brain moving. You can actually revisit these four questions any time you need to in the course of your life, to help think through any major decision.

For me, the urge to keep climbing the corporate ladder fizzled out when my division was sold. I was only 30, which meant I had 35 years of struggle ahead of me before I could retire- if I was lucky. Brad, on the other hand, made the decision that he wanted to retire at age 50, so he and his financial planner had been working on that model since his early twenties. I was not (and still am not) that level of a planner, so while I had all the retirement accounts set up, I'd never really thought about them. Wealth was obviously not a motivating factor for me. I was sick of the stress of an office job and a routine, so I would've answered "c" to the first question, and "b" to the second.

As for the other changes I put on hold due to fear? Too many to list! I am a very anxious person by nature, raised by two highly risk-averse individuals, married to someone who is sensible enough to have started investing at age 20. I am very good at being too afraid to change anything. In fact, I've had anxiety about wearing a different pair of socks while hiking, because the last time I changed my socks, something bad happened.

But that question- "is it really better to wait?"- kept haunting me.

At the end of the day, you are the only person in the entire world who can answer that question. There are compelling reasons on all sides of the argument, and there may be times when it is legitimately best to wait a bit. I suggest you make a list to help you figure out the pros and cons and any other angles that might appear. I recommend keeping a running list of thoughts over a period of time- perhaps a week, minimum.

In my case, I was definitely emotionally and physically prepared to leave the office behind, but not at all aware of the challenges that awaited me by starting a new career, working for myself, by myself, in a tiny blue van. Brad walked away from his desk with the three framed pictures he'd brought in and a heart full of ambition. His surprise came when the emotional and psychological aspects of being alone demonstrated that he was virtually "stranded" in his chosen work environment.

One or all of these intimidating concepts will arise over the next few years, perhaps together or individually. You may worry about being alone. You may become concerned that you'll do the same crummy task over and over for the rest of your life. Living from payment to payment may be a very real experience. You will frequently wonder if you have done the right thing.

But at the end of the day, will you regret it? I can't tell you the answer to that question, but for what it's worth, I haven't encountered anyone yet who does!

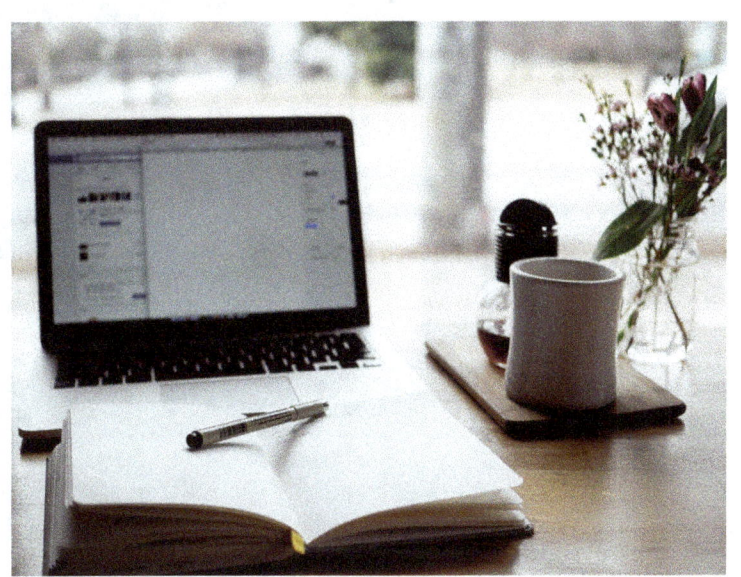

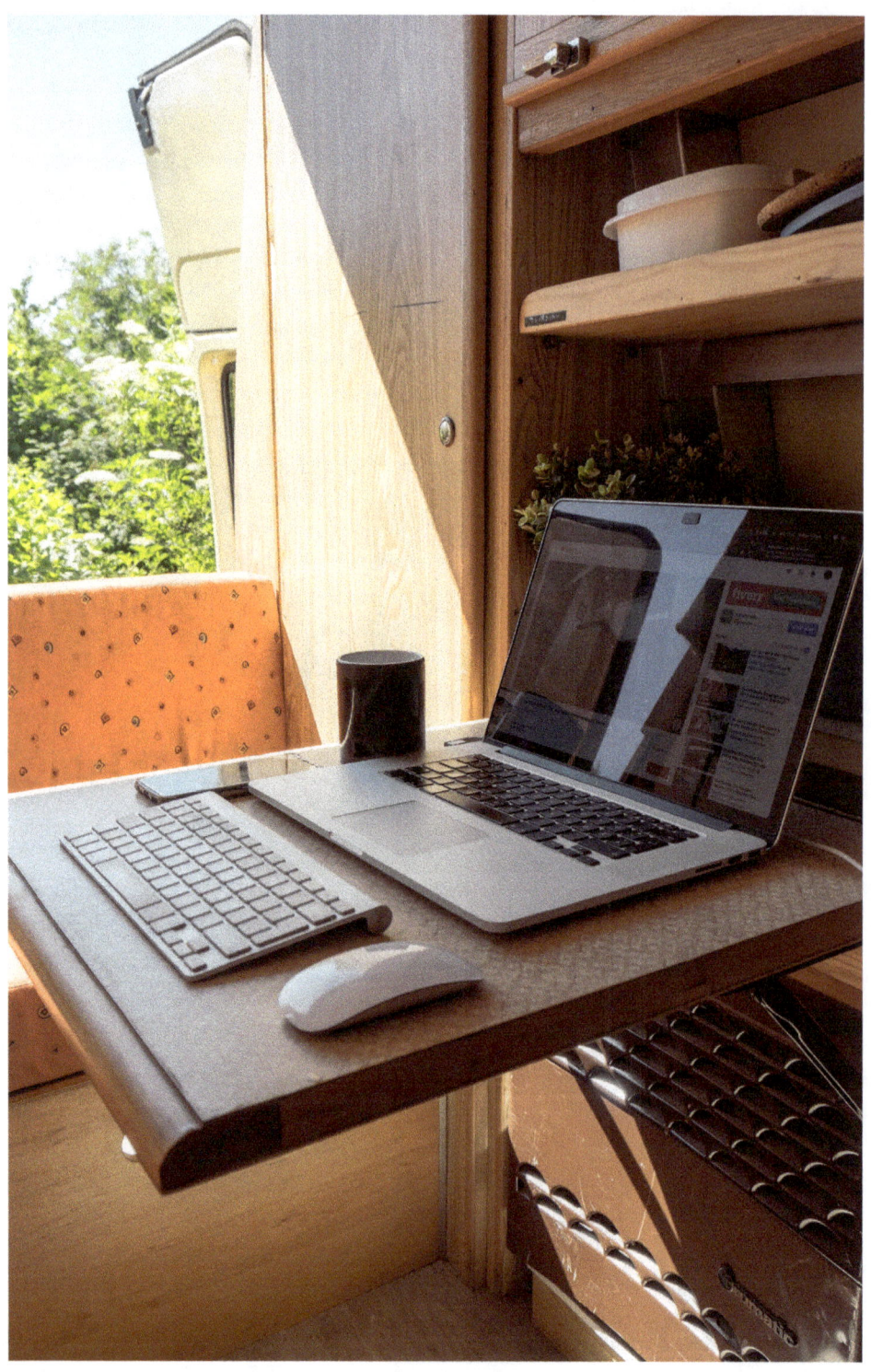

## Section Six: Wrapping It All Up

I would love to be able to end this book by telling you that if you follow these tips, you'll be a millionaire, living your best life in the near future. But that's just not realistic for all of us.

My goal with the various exercises presented throughout this book was to help you get into the right mindset for taking your profession out of the office and into your own life. Thanks to technological advances and the connectivity provided by the internet, the possibilities today are far greater than they were just ten years ago. Corporate workers can attend meetings virtually. Freelancers can connect with an infinite number of clients located all over the world. Side-hustlers and crafters can advertise their wares to the entire planet by creating a simple website. Even day-by-day workers can find employment in the next town they plan to visit by conducting a quick search on their phones.

Finding a gig via the internet may be easier than ever, but maintaining that employment through all of life's changes can be difficult. No matter what type of occupation you pursue, your own personal situation will find a way to interrupt. In some cases, that's a temporary blip that can be accommodated by minor adjustments in your current career situation. In other cases, that interruption will lead to the discovery of a brand new lifestyle!

If I had been told at the start of my professional life- fresh out of college in 2002- that in a matter of years I'd be writing books in the back of a van, I probably would have believed it, but assumed the worst. Chris Farley's "Saturday Night Live" motivational speaker character, Matt Foley, cautioned my generation time and time again about the perils of "living in a van down by the river." I probably would have interpreted that fate as a warning, rather than the extremely positive, fulfilling scenario that plays out my life.

And yet, here I am, lucky enough to do my two most favorite things every single day: explore and write. I'll be the first to admit that it hasn't been smooth sailing the whole time. The van breaks down from time to time. I have had several dozen panic attacks accompanied by unseemly banshee-level shrieking when the WiFi connection disappears right before a major deadline. On one particularly quaint occasion, the van broke down, the generator stopped, and the water line broke. We were able to get out of that mess within a few hours thanks to some very kind fellow boondockers, but the life lesson learned from that is that the worst case scenario is not just possible, it's plausible!

I hope to leave you feeling well-prepared and encouraged about the transition to working remotely. There is never a wrong time to do the exercises recommended. My experience in corporate human resources has demonstrated the value of revisiting these types of questions from time to time.

The days of stagnating in the same job for 30 continuous years have passed. While it's certainly admirable, we now live in a world of opportunity and development. Whether you choose to grow in your current role, or try different things for the rest of your life, "variety" and "flexibility" are now two of the most treasured qualities in an employee.

This may not be the last time you consider your job and think, "am I really doing the right thing? Am I happy here?" I encourage you to think of this transition not as a final place to rest, but another step towards the next big change, all of which are set along the path towards living your best possible life.

For your convenience, I have rounded up the main questions asked throughout this text, so you can refer to them whenever you like. You might want to hang this list up in a conspicuous place, or use it as journalling fodder. However you get to these answers is perfectly fine, as long as you're honest with yourself!

*Why do I want to work remotely?*

*How did I come to this potential decision?*

*What are some things I want to control?*

*What are some areas where I need more flexibility?*

*What are the pros and cons of working remotely?*

*What will I accomplish with this change?*

*Am I willing/able to take my current job on the road?*

*Am I interested in changing my career?*

*What are my talents, interests, and strong skills?*

*In my wildest dreams, what does my work/life balance look like?*

*How do I think this is going to work?*

*Who can I count on in my network?*

*How will I create my work space?*

*Do I have access to everything I need to get the job done?*

*What kind of schedule will work best for both my work and my lifestyle?*

*How do I inspire my own productivity?*

*What types of distractions might I encounter?*

*How do I work?*

*How important is the social aspect of your current work environment?*

*Where do you see yourself in ten years?*

*Do your expenses and income line up adequately?*

*Is it better to wait?*

----------------

This is likely to be a very exciting and nerve wrecking time for you. You will likely experience many emotions and have many thoughts racing through your head. You might lose sleep as you try to organize your thoughts. There will be anxiety at the great unknown that lies ahead, but also great relief as you manage to capture more and more control over your work/life balance.

For everyone reading this, I wish you a smooth transition. I urge you to stay confident even when you're completely broken down on a Colorado mountainside. I strongly believe that our experiences shape us, and that what we consider "failure" is just another type of experience telling us we were heading down the wrong path.

To aid you on your quest, I've included a section of resources that I have found helpful and that have been recommended to me by others who have left the office to seek a greater purpose.

Read on, and may you find the footholds that you need to reach greatness!

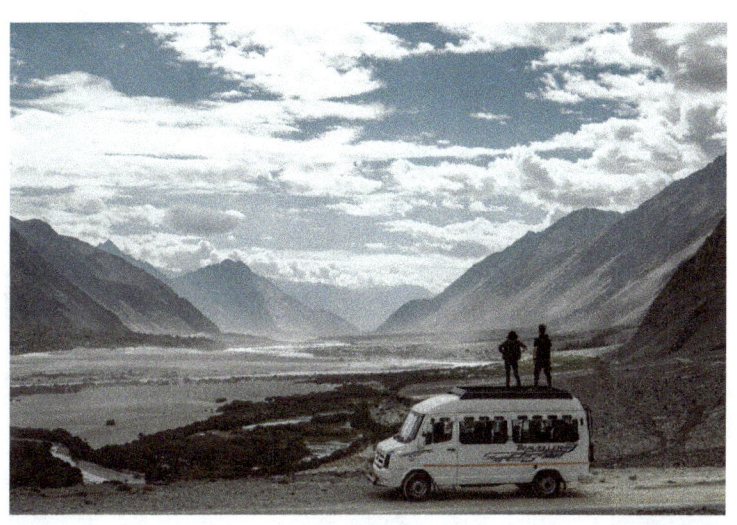

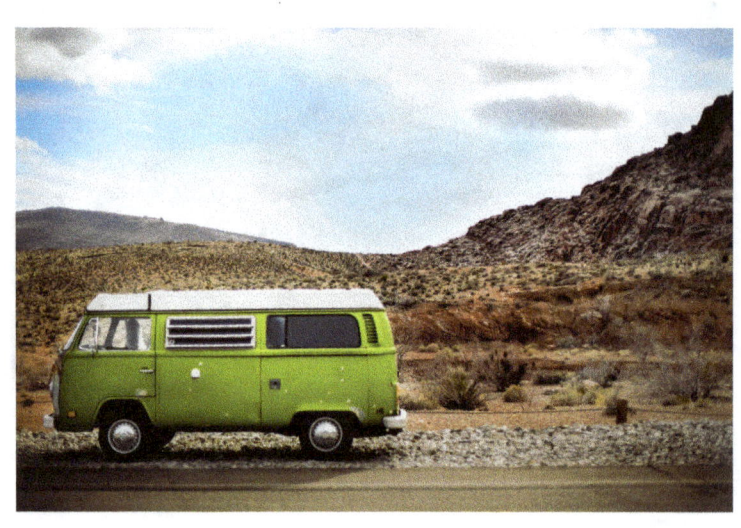

## Section 6: Resources for Former Office Workers

I've included a few links to sites that could potentially help you find the direction you'd like to go in creating the ultimate work location and situation for yourself. There also are links to groups and organizations that should provide support with the potential challenges mentioned earlier, including the social, financial, productivity-vs-distractions aspects, as well as tips to create a practical physical and emotional space for your new work environment.

None of these links are intended to be considered endorsements, and may not reflect the opinions of those affiliated with this book. These sites were cultivated merely for the possible assistance they can provide to those who are looking to make huge maneuvers in their professional lives. This list is not exhaustive, either- instead, think of it as a launching pad for the things you wish to learn about in greater detail!

### Productivity Management Resources

As mentioned several times, a change in work environment can impact your productivity. If you're the type who needs direct guidance to stay on task, or wouldn't mind a frequent reminder of due dates, appointments, and more, consider adding one of these resources to your daily structure.

My Life Organized: https://www.mylifeorganized.net/
Available for: iOS and Android, Windows
What it does: If you're the type of person who craves micromanagement, and whose "To Do" list looks more like the outline for a scholarly research paper, you might be the type to appreciate My Life Organized. This app breaks down all of your duties into tasks, all of your tasks into sub-tasks, and all of your lists into errands.

RescueTime: https://www.rescuetime.com/
Available for: iOS and Android
What it does: This app can be considered a Time Management or Productivity assistant, but really, it's an internet babysitter. RescueTime works in the background, keeping track of your internet behavior. If you're the

type who easily falls down internet rabbit holes, this is a way to keep you focused on your new goals, rather than getting distracted.

Timely: https://memory.ai/timely
Available for: iOS and Android, Mac and Windows
What it does: Timely is an AI app that pays attention to what you're doing so that it can learn how to be your ultimate productivity manager. It keeps track of your behaviors and tasks and creates schedules to help optimize your time. If you need help with accountability and staying on track with multiple projects, this type of AI app can be of assistance.

Toggl: https://toggl.com/
Available for: iOS, Mac, Android
What it does: Toggl is a time-tracking app that helps you see where you're spending the most of your time. It provides weekly, monthly, or annual reports to help you refocus on your time and efforts. This is helpful for anyone who wanders off chasing butterflies a bit too often!

Trello: https://trello.com/
Available for: iOS and Android, Mac and Windows
What it does: Trello is a visuals-based project management program. Think Pinterest, but instead of losing valuable hours adding things to your board, it helps you create a visual display of what you need to accomplish. This can help you maximize your efforts without added stress.

**Money Management Resources**
Whether you're making the full plunge to a new career or side-hustle, or you just want to stay on top with the changes that occur when you lose the long commute and wardrobe budget, these resources can help. The financial aspect of any change is something that truly has an impact on our lifestyles, whether we like it or not. If you're like me and struggle with anything more than basic math, consider a money management resource to keep you organized and apprised of your finances. Again, I'm not affiliated with any of these, but share them as popular options that exist.

Mint: https://www.mint.com/

Mint helps you keep track of all of your bills, all of your balances, and even your credit score from one central location. If you have memories of your parents spreading all of the bills, bank statements, and checks across the kitchen table once a month, consider all of that, only on one simple screen.

The Penny Hoarder: https://www.thepennyhoarder.com/

If you have a question that even potentially might impact your pocketbook, The Penny Hoarder probably has a few articles that can provide advice and guidance, covering a wide variety of topics that can help you understand where your money comes from and where it goes.

The Simple Dollar: https://www.thesimpledollar.com/blog-overview/

The key word in the title is "Simple." This blog is highly educational, especially for those who are taking control of their money in a new way. From scouting the best insurance products, to helping you understand how you can make your savings work for you, this blog covers it all.

Stacking Benjamins: https://www.stackingbenjamins.com/about/

This is a podcast, but a valuable resource. Whether you tune in while you drive your van into the sunset, or in your headphones during a break, there's a wide variety of very relatable financial discussions for nearly every person's situation

Wally: https://www.wally.me/

Wally is for visual learners. It provides users with options to track expenses, create and maintain a budget, organizes receipts and other financial documents, and can even help synchronize family expenses and earnings.

**Technical Resources**

I've divided this section up into "Home Office" and "Working on the Run," because while there is some overlap between the two scenarios, you likely won't have any trouble with WiFi installation in a home that doesn't have wheels and a motor. These resources range from workspaces to wires, and help with a lot of the "where" and "how can I" questions that might arise when setting up your new workspace.

For those who will be working from an office that doesn't move, here are a few helpful links:

Decor and Space Tips:
https://www.thespruce.com/how-to-set-up-a-workable-home-office-1977403
https://www.hgtv.com/design/rooms/other-rooms/10-tips-for-designing-your-home-office

Both The Spruce and HGTV.com are absolute rabbit holes of gorgeous design ideas and amazing aesthetics, but these practical articles are a good place to get started if you're not sure how to proceed.

Ergonomics:
https://www.mayoclinic.org/healthy-lifestyle/adult-health/in-depth/office-ergonomics/art-20046169
https://ergo-plus.com/workplace-ergonomics/

You may not realize it right now, but your office set up, including your desk, chair, keyboard, mousepad, and monitor are all set up to help you avoid long and short term pain. Your transition to a new work space should not need to coincide with an increase in chiropractic and massage expenses. Check out these tips to ensure you're in the best form possible.

For Those Working For Themselves:
https://www.thebalancesmb.com/setting-up-home-office-845850

The Balance Small Business has plenty of tips for new freelancers, side-hustlers, and small business owners. This particular article includes some interesting tips for creating a workspace... which you can then follow to other tips you might need.

For Parents:
https://hbr.org/2017/03/balancing-parenting-and-work-stress-a-guide

https://www.parents.com/parenting/work/life-balance/
https://www.forbes.com/working-remote/#30f3de8e413f
https://www.forbes.com/forbeswomen/#29642e41621e

I realize this topic wasn't touched on much throughout the course of the book, but not because I didn't feel it deserves attention. There are so many considerations regarding children, parenting, homeschooling, activities, and more that the topic deserves its own book. These are just a small sample of some of the resources my friends who are parents have mentioned. You may also wish to network with other parents through LinkedIn, Facebook groups and blogs, as the community effort is strong.

And if you're hitting the road soon, take a look at these offerings:
Connectivity:
https://www.opensignal.com/
https://faroutride.com/internet-vanlife/
https://www.chasingthewildgoose.com/vanlife-wifi-options/
https://vanliving101.com/2019/09/30/create-your-own-secured-wifi-hotspot-in-your-van/

The first link is a helpful map that I found a little too late for my own benefit, which is why I share it here. Open Signal can help you figure out where you can get a cellphone and WiFi signal, based on your carrier. This is the type of information you should consult before you plan a day of wandering, especially if you have a deadline creeping up.

The other three links are expert Van Lifer accounts of different ways you can access WiFi on the road.

Please note: Technology changes every day. These links are contemporary to the publication of this book, and may or may not be helpful at the time of your specific voyage.

Putting an Office in Your Van:
https://www.parkedinparadise.com/mobile-office/
https://www.youtube.com/watch?v=5JEN5zcnc40

https://pursuitist.com/office-on-wheels-for-those-who-love-to-work-on-the-go/
https://www.technicallywizardry.com/mobile-office-desk-van/

Ultimately, how you fit your office into your van, skoolie, RV, or camper is going to depend on the space you have, your carpentry and creating skills, and your overall grand plan. I wanted to provide a few links to those who have done it, though, so you can gain inspiration and rest assured that it can be done.

Recommended Reading For Making It Work:
http://thevanual.com/working-and-living/
https://divineontheroad.com/van-life-remote-jobs/
https://www.outsideonline.com/2316796/i-gave-my-house-vanlife-while-holding-down-9-5
https://marcysutton.com/remote-work-van-life

It may seem strange that I'm including other people's blogs in my book, but #VanLife isn't just a lifestyle, it's a community. I wanted to take the opportunity to demonstrate that there are other people who do this, and to provide you with the chance to get their perspective on the matter. Again, I couldn't include links to every single Van Lifer's thoughts on the matter, but I encourage anyone considering this to read anything they can from people who have been there and done that. Don't just take my word for it!

### Network/Community Resources

Maintaining community is a strong instinct within human nature, and one that we use to our advantage. We crave the support and interaction of sympathetic parties. These sites are designed to help motivate remote workers, and alleviate some of the growing pains by connecting you with others who are wandering down similar paths.

I'd also like to mention that LinkedIn, Facebook, and Reddit are all great community resources for multiple reasons. Forums are not without opinions of course, so join discussions at your own risk, but the "real people talking about real things" model is something that has helped many people feel comfortable with their challenges and not so alone.

I've tried to include a little something for everyone here, since we touched on many different scenarios in the course of the book.

For Women:
Power to Fly: https://powertofly.com/
Remote Woman: https://remotewoman.com/community/
TED for Women: https://www.ted.com/topics/women+in+business
Women Entrepreneur: https://www.entrepreneur.com/women
It pains me to say it, but even today, women are met with a different set of challenges in the workforce. These sites provide connections to jobs, to resources to support and guide, and access to a community of women who face similar situations.

For Side Hustlers:
Believe In A Budget: https://believeinabudget.com/
Side Hustle Nation: https://www.facebook.com/groups/sidehustlenation/
Side Hustle School: https://sidehustleschool.com/
All of these represent useful tools for getting started with your side hustle. I've included some blogs, some podcasts, some training tools, and idea generators. Again, not an exhaustive list, but certainly one that should get the brain focused on making this happen!

For Freelancers:
Freelance Lift: https://www.freelancelift.com/
Freelancers' Union: https://www.freelancersunion.org/
The Middle Finger Project Blog: https://www.themiddlefingerproject.org/blog/
One Woman Shop- A Solopreneur Community and Resource Hub: https://onewomanshop.com/
Again, there are thousands of resources for freelancers to join minds with other freelancers. I wanted to include a few blogs and communities to allow a variety of points of view on this topic. Each of these links leads to plenty of thoughts, opinions, experiences, and regular daily commentary

on the reality of freelancing, along with valuable resources for those of us living the dream.

For Corporate Workers:
Virtual Vocations: https://www.virtualvocations.com/blog/
The Remote Work Summit: https://www.theremoteworksummit.com/
Work Remotely: https://slofile.com/slack/workremotely
Remote Work Slack: https://remoteworkslack.com/?ref=workfrom.co/chat
While it may not be exactly the same as doing shots at the bar within walking distance of the office, these communities, blogs, and resources can help re-energize the social needs within you. Plus, you'll get the chance to banter, vent, bemoan, and learn without a hefty bar bill.

For Those Working from the Road:
Project Van Life Forum: https://forum.projectvanlife.com/
Vanlife Magazine Forum: https://vanlifemagazine.co/
The Vanlife App: https://www.thevanlifeapp.com/
Kristine Hudson's Facebook Group: https://www.facebook.com/eternal-vantrip/
These are just a few of the online communities available for folks, including my own fledgling Facebook community. While these forums cover a variety of topics relevant to anyone who's home has wheels, work, productivity, and money are definitely amongst those topics. Plus, if you don't see what you need to know, start a thread!

If you know of a good link, resource, or helpful community, feel free to share it on my official Facebook page. After all, you're never alone!

TIPS AND TRICKS FOR A HEALTHY VAN LIFESTYLE

# FROM WHEELS TO WELLNESS

Kristine Hudson

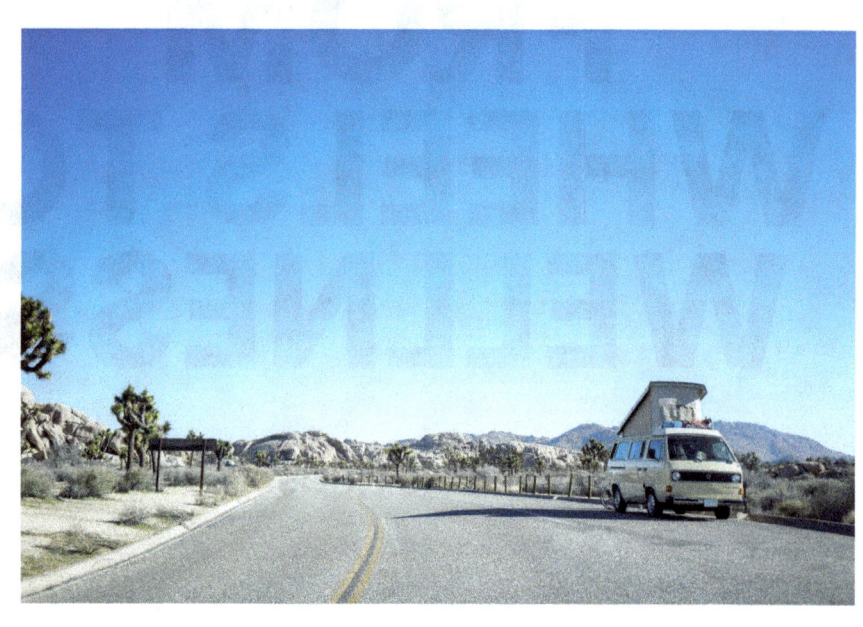

## Section 1: Introduction

If you're reading this book, chances are pretty good that you're either knee-deep in van life or preparing to embark on the greatest adventure of your life. After all, the topic of maintaining your health and wellness while living on the road is a pretty niche topic.

But this book is intended not just for van lifers, but for roadtrippers, frequent fliers, and anyone whose lifestyle lacks routine, ordinariness, or regularity. This is the 21st century; technology has made a lot of previously unimaginable things very possible.

For example, living on the road is no longer for "hobos and nomads," as my grandmother was fond of saying. Van life is accessible to many people; it's become a way of life for more individuals than ever before. Whether they are living on the road full-time, or taking every possible opportunity to roam, more and more people are packing up their families, their pets, and their jobs to make a home on wheels.

It's not just the #VanLife crowd, either. While some like to "blame" the Millennial penchant for wanderlust for the sudden renewed interest in traveling to all ends of the Earth, the truth is that humans have always loved travel. Many of us are exercising this innate need to roam and choose to broaden our horizons by learning more about the places and people that make up this beautiful planet.

And so here you are, ready to immerse yourself in new experiences through previously uncharted territory. You've probably considered so many things and made so many decisions, but honestly, the process is just starting. A life on the road- whether a permanent situation or a small dose of freedom - requires making a lot of choices on the fly:

> "Do I stop for gas now, or hope I can make it to the next town?"
> "Should I take the loop trail clockwise or counter-clockwise?"
> "Can I fit in a three-mile bike ride before my next conference call?"

These questions are just a sample of the regular thoughts from any traveler's day.

Therefore, it stands to reason that some things are going to fall by the wayside. One of the most common things people forget when traveling – besides their toothpaste – is to take care of themselves physically, psychologically, and even preventively. It's really easy to get swept up in the day-to-day of just experiencing things, and forget about some of the more mundane aspects of existence.

When we live in a stationary home, we regularly get reminders about that sort of thing. The dentist sends a cheerful postcard to remind us to stop by. Doctors call to confirm your appointments 24 hours ahead of time. Commercials for your favorite brand of vitamins remind you to add them to the grocery list. There's a sense of order that comes with domesticity.

But then you hit the road. Days stop having names and numbers. It's a blur of places, things, experiences, and emotions, and you honestly can't remember what you had for dinner two nights ago, much less whether you took your vitamins. And are you squinting because of the sun, or because it's been two years since your last eye exam?

These things catch up with us quickly, and if there's one thing people on the road "ain't got time for," it's being out of commission due to illness or injury. From nasty viruses and mental malaise to breaks and sprains, it doesn't take much to take you out of the game when you're traveling.

I wrote this guide as a gentle reminder for everyone on the road to take care of themselves. If there's one thing we have learned during the COVID-19 crisis, it's that disease travels faster than we do. Despite anyone's best intentions, you can never be too cautious about health and wellness.

My van life journey started in 2018, before masks and social distancing became part of the experience. Even then, my husband Brad and I were surprised at how devastating even a simple cold could be to our lifestyle. To write this book, I've worked with other van lifers and folks within the health and medical communities - from nurses and pediatricians to physical therapists and nutritionists - who shared tips, experiences, and ideas related to maintaining your own wellness while doing some serious traveling.

While I can't promise that you'll live forever without a single sniffle after reading this book, I am fairly confident that you'll gain a few ideas that can help you improve your overall outlook on wellness. My goal is simply to point out some of the challenges that we might encounter on the road, in the wild, or anytime we abandon ourselves to a less domesticated lifestyle, and to equip you with a few pointers to confront those obstacles with practical solutions.

Whether you use this book as a launching pad for a daily health regimen or as a reminder to refill your first aid kit, consider the information in this book, as well as the resources at the end, as a reference for whenever you find yourself in a state of adventuring. After all, there's never a bad time to practice healthy habits!

## Chapter 1: What You Need to Know

There are germs literally everywhere. I'm not telling you this because you don't know it. Companies that market cleaning products spend billions of dollars each year to make sure we all know it. I'm mentioning this here within the context of this book because all of the little particles of bacteria, viruses, molds, and fungi that you meet on a doorknob in New Orleans, at a gas station in Topeka, or even at a campsite in Colusa, are more than happy to move into your van and tag along on your adventures. Science moment: most bacteria and viruses don't live on surfaces as long as they do in a host because their ability to reproduce is compromised. However, there are always exceptions. A lot of rhinoviruses, one of the organisms behind the common cold, can remain on your hands in an infectious state for hours. Methicillin-resistant Staphylococcus aureus - better known by its street name, MRSA – can hang out on surfaces for weeks, just waiting for a nice open wound to start infecting your body.

Now, my goal here isn't to scare you into never leaving the van again. The point I'm trying to make is that there are different types of bacteria, viruses, molds, and fungi everywhere, and you're going to encounter them no matter what. When you live in a van or have a very travel-forward lifestyle, you're going to be taking your hands everywhere you go. They'll meet all sorts of new germs, and they may even be responsible for introducing new flora and fauna to new areas… if you don't take precautions.

Again, this isn't supposed to be scary, just a little bit of common-sense. You've probably been through this experience on a smaller scale whenever you start a new job, your child returns to school, or you take the whole family on a vacation; within a week or two, everyone in your household gets sick with the same thing. It's very common though, and usually not devastating. Your body getting sick is how it trains itself to make antibodies that protect you the next time you encounter that particular strain of germ.

As travelers, we live by the phrase "take nothing but pictures; leave nothing but footprints." So, we're automatically responsible for not starting a wave of infection in the places we visit. Many indigenous people were wiped out when new diseases were brought to their homelands. Even though the difference between Indiana and Iowa today may not seem great, the idea of getting an entire community sick because we happened to stop at a gas station at the same time is more guilt than I personally can handle.

The magnitude of our impact is more than we can measure, so as van lifers, we need to be aware of our own actions. Not just for the health and wellness of everyone in our van, but for the communities we visit too.

In this book, we'll look at ways to nurture a healthy lifestyle in and out of the van. I am not going to give you diet ideas or weight loss or weight training tips. I'm not going to tell you what combination of essential oils will cure dysentery. What I am going to do is remind you of all the things that might fall by the wayside when you leave domesticity behind. If the last few paragraphs have had any impact on you, you shouldn't be surprised when I say the number one thing you need to do on the road, no matter what, is **wash your hands!**

Let's expand on that. Let's take a look at not just how you can reduce the spread of disease, but how you can take care of yourself no matter where you are. Everything from preventive care to keep yourself well, to supplies every van lifer should have on hand, to nutrition and exercise tips, mental health considerations, and even what you can do to reduce your own germy footprints will make an appearance in the following pages.

Consider this book a handy helper to remind you to take care of yourself no matter where you're going. If you haven't left the stationary home yet, some of this might seem obvious. But once you answer the call of the wild and hit the road, you may find that you become a bit... well, feral, for lack of a better term. My goal is to create a few "oh yeah" moments to keep your mind and body on track for staying healthy no matter what sort of shenanigans you're enjoying!

## Chapter 2: What Do I Know?

So if I'm writing a book about health and wellness, I must be a doctor, right? I'm not. Though I worked in close proximity with doctors for years as a human resources consultant within the health and wellness division of an insurance company, that hardly counts as medical credentials.

An amusing truth is that everyone in my family is either a healthcare worker or an engineer. I'm the "black sheep" writer, but this actually works in my favor. Whenever something stops working correctly - whether it's me or something in my home - I have someone to call. And whenever they need their resumes updated, they call me. It's a reciprocal relationship!

When I was packing for my first van excursion, I had a panel of experts to explain exactly why I needed to pack acetaminophen, ibuprofen, and naproxen (it has to do with the way each provides relief for fevers and inflammation, if you're wondering). Not everyone has access to that type of support, so I wanted to share what I could, when I could, to help any other van newbies who are standing in similar shoes, wondering what's enough.

Two years on the road leaves you with plenty of experiential knowledge too. I'm not here to share weird tips and tricks that may or may not be medically sound, but practical things you wish someone would tell you. Like, "pack way more towels than you think you need." Think of this book as a favorite uncle, giving you a few pointers from hard-earned experience.

While not all of the advice in this book is anecdotal, I am going to tell quite a few stories. One thing that I did not fully realize until I started living in a van is that I am clumsy. I lack balance, grace, and coordination on an almost amusing level. As a result, many of the things I have learned about keeping the body well come from orthopedists, sports physicians, and physical therapists I've met along the way. These trained professionals have listened to my complaints and helped me come up with van-friendly ways to keep my battered body functioning, despite my best efforts. I'm not trying to take the place of these experts, but instead share what they wish they could tell everyone in my shoes.

The topic of mental health is also near and dear to me. Like many people in the United States, I struggle with anxiety and depression. This is something I have been working on since I first came into the realization that I was not okay in 1999. I'm not an expert, just someone who is acutely aware of how being on the road can do strange things to not just your body, but your mind. The section about mental health isn't just going to be a list of what I do, but more of a collection of recommendations I've learned from working very closely with mental healthcare providers and others on the road.

If you are ready for help right now, here are some immediate resources:
- The 24/7 helpline for Substance Abuse and Mental Health Services

Administration is 1-800-662-HELP (4357).
- Lifeline for National Suicide Prevention can be reached at 1-800-273-8255.

Both of these numbers provide free, confidential connection to individuals and services that can help you. You can also find more information in the Resources section.

Finally, I don't want anyone to think that I'm a health snob or a wellness know-it-all. I have never had a kale smoothie, and I sometimes forget my sunblock. If anything, think of this book as a good friend or worldly relative coming up to you before you leave for the road and saying, "Hey, let me tell you about a bunch of stuff I didn't think of. Here's how they came to be a problem, and here's what I learned about it." Take what you will. I'm not going to make medical recommendations. I am going to share stories about the cringe-worthy lessons my husband and I have learned about health and wellness on the open road. I'm definitely going to tell you about the time I fell off a cliff (and hopefully you'll laugh as much as I did).

Don't consider this book a byway for actual medical advice. I'm not diagnosing anything or recommending a course of treatment. I am, however, going to tell you to wash your hands; in fact, I'll mention it frequently. And while you're at it, your laundry, your van, your produce, and… well, just read on.

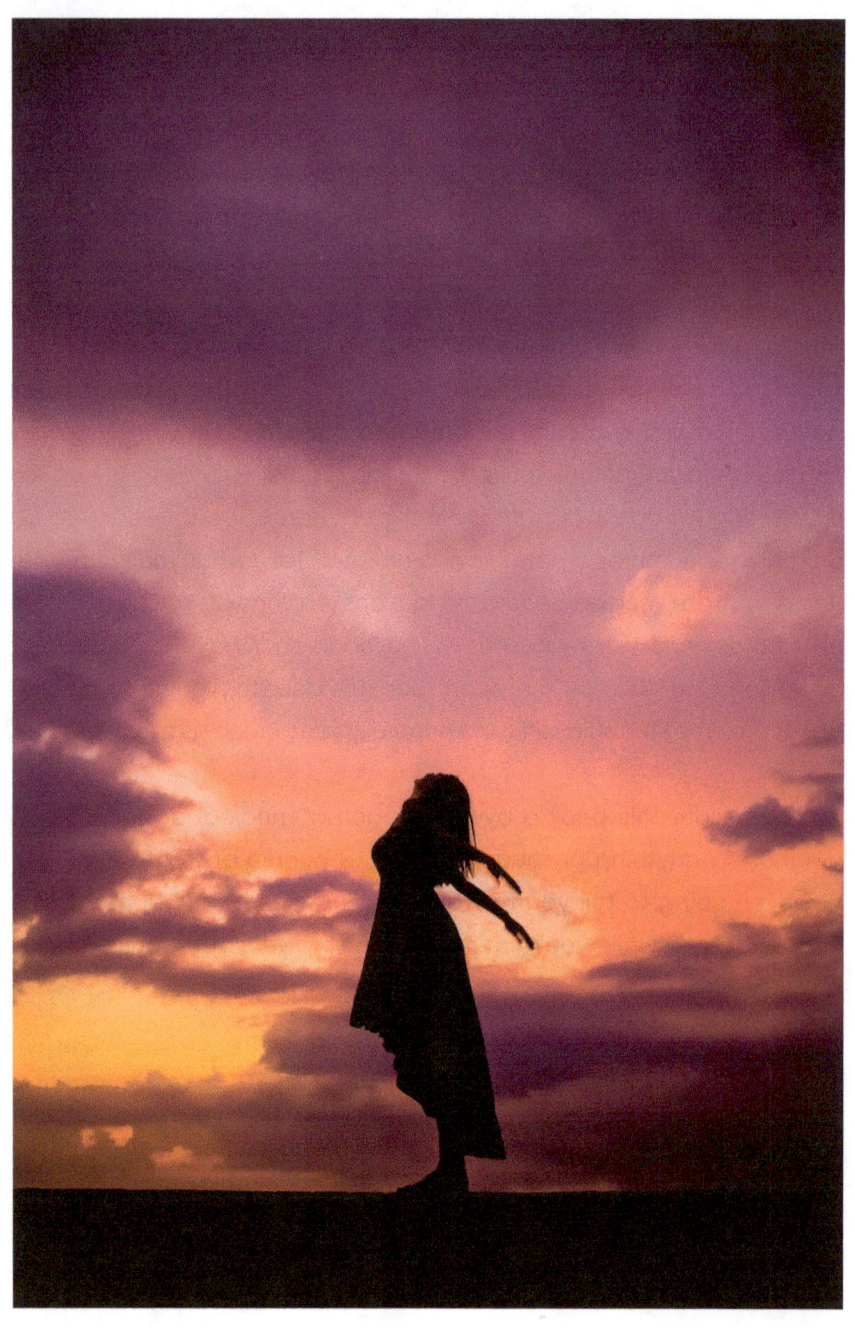

## Section 2: Taking Care of Your One and Only Body

You've probably heard the phrase "You've only got one body!" While it's typically thrown about in an annoying diet campaign, there's no denying the truth of the statement. In fact, there's nothing that validates the phrase quite like choosing to live a nomadic lifestyle in a van.

At least, that's what was running through my mind when I battled a fever and tonsillitis somewhere in Upstate New York. Our first tour of the United States was winding down, and I was torn between trying to power through hiking the Adirondacks or sleeping until I felt better. I felt so crummy, I actually cried. I desperately wanted to feel great and do all the things I dreamed of doing. "I may never get this chance again!" my brain wailed. "Yes, but you've only got one body," shot back my throat, raging with infection.

I share this experience because we're often very stubborn when it comes to our overall physical health. Most of us know how to eat well, brush our teeth, and exercise regularly. These are all great habits to maintain and will do a lot to keep you healthy in the long run. But let's take a few things out of the equation. For example, let's say you have limited access to running water. You have no idea where the closest grocery store is. You have extremely limited refrigeration, and there's definitely not a treadmill in sight.

Van life is full of sacrifices - many of which are made gleefully - but your health should not be one of the choices on the table. You may not have considered the impact of van life on seemingly insignificant activities like brushing your teeth. However, it only takes one day without running water to realize how much we take these things for granted. Even the act of getting up at midnight for a quick trip to the bathroom can become challenging when your home has four wheels (and no toilet).

So, let's take a look at some of the things you can do to proactively keep that one and only magnificent body of yours in top condition while on the road. You may still miss some of the convenience of having a stationary kitchen and bathroom, but you don't have to sacrifice overall wellness!

## Chapter 1: Keeping Up with Preventive Care

Preventive care is an umbrella term for taking care of your body each and every day to prevent future illnesses. The concept is obvious: if you take care of your body, you will be rewarded with wellness. Granted, preventive care isn't going to take care of every possibility. The human body is vast, complex, and does a lot of weird things when we least expect it. Just as you have packed your van to be prepared for whatever comes your way, practicing regular preventive care is the best way to do the same for your body.

The following preventive care guidelines are all equally important, so please don't view this as a definitive ranking of what to do. Instead, consider all of these as reminders that even though you're living a "wild and free" lifestyle, every body has limitations.

**The Steps to Preventive Care**
The first recommendation I'd like to share is to **Get Checked Out.** While no one understands the experience of living in your body as well as you do, you can easily be unaware of some of the finer details of your existence. Therefore, it's a great idea to visit a general practitioner, dentist, and optometrist (eye-doctor) on a regular basis.

I know what you're thinking, believe me. No one really enjoys going for a physical or dental exam. It's time-consuming, it almost always results in bad news and anxiety, it's expensive, and in some cases, painful. Even if the doctor helpfully offers a lollipop after everything is said and done, our adult brains aren't sure that what we've endured was worth it.

The truth is that regular examinations are one of the simplest ways to maintain good health. When you go in for a standard physical, your doctor will check your weight, blood pressure, and check your breathing and heart rate. They may also run some biometric blood work to measure cholesterol, and blood sugar. While this may seem like a giant waste of time to people who are regularly active and in good health, here's the bottom line: **most of the time, we don't know what's wrong unless we know what's right.**

By receiving regular physical examinations, you'll get to know your baseline levels – what "healthy" looks like for your body. That way, when something does feel bad, you'll be able to compare it to what "good" feels like for you.

Additionally, visiting a doctor regularly provides the opportunity to find early warning signs of potential health problems. The more data you have regarding your own health, the easier it will be to catch any inconsistencies that could become a much larger obstacle down the road.

The same goes for dental exams. Practicing regular dental health is relatively simple, even in a van. We'll dive into some additional tips on how to work oral hygiene into a world without running water later in this book, but brushing and flossing regularly is the first step in keeping your teeth and gums healthy. It's also a great idea to visit a dentist at least once a year to thoroughly check for cavities, signs of disease, and other problems that you might not be able to see or diagnose on your own.

Last, but certainly not least, are eye exams. Millions of people around the world rely on corrective lenses of some sort. Contrary to the teasing we may have received in elementary school, wearing glasses is a fantastic idea for those with less than perfect vision. Straining to see properly can cause a lot of wear and tear on the eyes and result in some pretty mind-blowing headaches.

Let's not be coy. If you're driving a van, you really should have your eyes checked for the safety of your passengers and everyone else on the road. Driving with impaired vision is really dangerous. From an adventurer's point of view, why on Earth would you want to explore the planet if you can barely see it?

So, when should you visit all of these medical practitioners? Well, experts don't entirely agree on frequency, but "at least once a year" seems to be the consensus. Younger people with low family history of risk or no pre-existing conditions can often get away with having a physical every three years. Children, those over 50, and anyone experiencing chronic conditions should visit more frequently.

Other wellness exams that are dependent on age, sex, and family history are also recommended. For example, all women should receive a Well Woman visit each year, and women over 40 should receive regular mammograms. Colonoscopies are recommended for adults over 50 or those with a family history of digestive tract issues.

In many cases, I might be preaching to the proverbial choir here. You might be well on board with preventive care, but you may simultaneously wonder how you're supposed to do all that from a van, RV, skoolie, or another free-wheeling home base.

There are a few options in this modern world! One rather recent advent is the walk-in clinic model. These walk-in style operations can be found in grocery stores and pharmacies, or as free-standing options for those who need simple and direct medical care. Often, you can visit any of these at any time during their open hours without an appointment or by calling ahead. They provide a variety of services, such as physical exams, vaccinations, and consultations. Generally speaking, you'll be in and out from your session very quickly, and at a low cost.

Surprisingly, vision exams can also be very simply arranged. Reputable eye care resources can be found in department stores and shopping malls. While eye appointments may need to be scheduled in advance, it's generally quite simple to find a nearby practice with an appointment available when scrolling through a quick online search via your smartphone.

Dental care can be a bit trickier because appointments tend to fill up quickly and may be hard to come by, unless you have a true dental emergency. If you have a dentist you know and love, you may wish to finagle your road trip so that you'll be in the neighborhood. This is actually my preferred method, because Brad and I are really, really bad about going to the dentist regularly. Brad just never got in the habit of going each year, and

I have an active terror of dentists (my apologies to anyone in the dental community- it's not you, it's me!). We found a patient and thorough dentist at our home base in Ohio. When we get our reminder texts from the practice, we make appointments, then get ready to loop back home for a few weeks. We get the opportunity to visit with our friends and family at home, and take care of that annual dentist visit in one swoop. In our case, we also throw in any other yearly check-ups as well.

Another option is to "plant" for a bit. In this case, you find a place to park for a few weeks and schedule any and all appointments to coincide with your time at that location. This can be helpful for any appointments that may have a potential follow-up, regardless of the type of practitioner you see. I have seen many traveling families utilize this option to ensure all the kids are able to see the doctor, dentist, and optometrist at once. Especially in cases where a doctor may have to order out for a prescription (or in the case of vision, order contacts or glasses for you), it can be easier to stay in one place for a bit. While some van dwellers may wince at the idea of staying in place for more than a few nights, remember this sacrifice is ultimately for your health and longevity!

Hand-in-hand with getting regular check-ups as part of your preventive care routine is vaccinations and booster shots. I know this is a super controversial topic, and I'm not going to spend time fanning the flames with discussion about whether you should or should not be vaccinated. I'll assume that, if you're reading this book, you are a grown adult with bodily autonomy who can make those decisions for yourself. If you are making decisions on behalf of your children, I hope that you do so with a full understanding of your family members' health and well-being.

I would also like to mention that a nomadic lifestyle has its own perils when it comes to spreading and contracting disease, as we van lifers come in contact with more people and more potential health threats than most people. Instead, we spend all of our time in an incubator on wheels, dragging all the fun viruses and bacteria we encounter along the way back to our van. While this book is filled with tips that can help mitigate becoming a modern day Typhoid Mary, there is significant scientific data that suggests that certain vaccines will help in this regard as well.

Additionally, if this is your first time living largely in the wilderness, you may want to consider potential environmental concerns that can be avoided with vaccinations. Clostridium bacteria, which causes Tetanus, are common in soil, dust, and manure deposits, all of which are very commonly found in the wilderness. This bacteria enters the body through even small cuts and impacts the central nervous system. Ultimately, untreated tetanus can lead to death by suffocation as muscles spasm and harden throughout the body.

Another consideration is rabies. Wild animals all over the United States can become infected by and transmit rabies, even though encountering a rabid animal in cities and suburbs is far less likely. When you're on the trail or boondocking, however, it's highly unlikely that an Animal Control official will roll up at exactly the right time to capture and remove the suffering animal. Instead, the best idea is to not come in direct contact with any wild animal you meet along the way, and consider getting a rabies vaccine before you hit the road.

Next on the preventive care checklist are your maintenance medications. Nearly half the population requires a daily dose of some type of medication, so if this is you, you're not alone. "Maintenance medication" refers to daily medication required for chronic conditions such as diabetes, asthma, arthritis, and many more.

The reason these drugs are so effective at helping people maintain wellness is because they are taken every day. This means a consistent amount of the drug is present to relieve certain symptoms. Without these drugs, individuals can experience a great deal of discomfort or potentially life-threatening symptoms. Therefore, it is important that anyone on a maintenance medication stay on a regular schedule.

There are two components to this: scheduling and refilling. Many of these drugs must be taken at the same time each day, while others need to be taken as symptoms present themselves. If you are on a daily schedule, there's one little, sneaky thing that happens as you travel - time zones. If you'll be going back and forth across time zones, make sure you discuss this with your doctor to avoid any unpleasant situations.

The thought of refilling your prescriptions while on the road can be intimidating. Personally, I'm on several daily medications for a slew of conditions, and I was genuinely afraid that I would have to return to Ohio every month to pick up my drugs. One of my doctors was an invaluable resource; she made sure I transferred all of my prescriptions to a national pharmacy chain. She also put a note on the prescription file that could be viewed through the pharmacy's system, explaining that I am traveling, and if I request my prescriptions in another state, it is valid. There were very few instances in which I wasn't able to waltz into the local chain and pick up my prescription. However, in those cases, the pharmacy staff very helpfully contacted my doctor, who was able to verify my prescription. All I had to do was present identification!

In many ways, picking up meds on the road was easier than at home. Many national chains have mobile apps, which help you find local pharmacies and request refills to specific locations. Just make sure you opt out of any automatic refills, or your prescription might be waiting for you to pick up several states away!

**A Few Words About Insurance**
The American concept of health, dental, and vision insurance is incredibly complicated. I should know - employee benefits was my area of expertise during my 10+ years in human resources. The concept is so complicated, in fact, I was hired as a personalized coach to explain health and welfare benefits to their employees. My main takeaway from that project was that health insurance has become nearly impossible for the everyday person to understand.

And to make matters worse, it's equally as difficult to survive in this country without health insurance. My goal is not to make this a whiny rant, but the facts speak for themselves. As a clumsy person, I once managed to slice my hand open while opening a $1 dog toy. What can I say? I'm talented. The resulting emergency room visit consisted of a nurse practitioner evaluating the wound, determining it could not be stitched due to its placement, giving me a special soap to keep it clean, and showing me how to bandage it to minimize the scar. As I was without insurance at the time, the visit resulted in a $1250 bill.

Naturally, I immediately regretted seeking medical attention. Amusingly enough, for my troubles of having to choose between paying rent and a medical bill for a few months, I still have no feeling in part of my finger. At least the scar is kind of cute!

Medical care is incredibly expensive. Health insurance is also very expensive, and incredibly confusing. So, what should you do?

My number one recommendation is to do the math. There are a lot of factors that go into determining whether or not you should have health insurance, and from there, what type of plan you should have.

First, consider your overall budget. What type of income will you be looking at in your van life scenario? Do you have a savings or checking account as a safety net?

Next, consider your overall health. Do you have any chronic conditions? Do you require maintenance prescriptions? Are you relatively healthy, but accident prone? One small detour to take in these considerations is to note what you plan to do while living in your van, and any potentially related risks to your health. Are you going to spend a lot of time driving, which could increase your chances of being in an automobile-related accident? Will you be doing a lot of hiking, climbing, or rappelling? Those are more risk factors to take into consideration.

A typical emergency room visit costs upwards of $1,000 without insurance, and visits to urgent care are generally in the low $100s to low $1,000s, depending on your reason for visiting. My visit to urgent care for having debris removed from my ear was around $300 without insurance. However, going to the emergency room after hours to assess my injuries after falling off of a cliff would have been around $8,000 without insurance. I meant it when I said I was accident prone – Brad and I actually accounted for me to have two medical emergencies each year when doing this exercise ourselves.

What we're gathering here are the numbers of "What You Can Afford" and "Anticipated Medical Costs." If you're pretty healthy, but your chances of falling off a cliff as I did are high, then you might want to include up to $10,000 for medical expenses. I got off lightly because I have my own crutches and air cast.

If you have regular prescriptions you must take, check out the price before and after insurance, if you're purchasing them with insurance right now. If you have regular medical appointments, add those to the total based on the rate you are currently billed AND what they would cost if you didn't have insurance.

You might benefit from making an easy chart like this:

| Expense | With Insurance | Without Insurance |
| --- | --- | --- |
| Daily Prescriptions | $35/month = $420 total | $550/month = $6,600 total |
| Appointment with Dr. Smith | $20 copay per visit<br>x 4 visits per year<br>$80 total | $165 per visit<br>x 4 visits per year<br>$660 total |
| Potential visit to urgent care (hypothetical) | $75 copay | $500 |
| Total Costs | $420 + $80 + $75 = $575 | $6,600 + $660 + $500 = $7,650 |

The annual total with insurance is calculated as:
$35 x 12= $420
$20 x 4 = $80
$420 + $80 + $75 = $575

We use the same process for the "without insurance" figures:
$550 x 12 = $6,600
$165 x 4 = $660
$6,600 + $660 + $500= $7,760

These numbers are actually based on my own medical usage, using my current insurance for the "with insurance" figures, and my experiences without insurance in 2017 for the "without insurance" figures. Your own expenses may vary greatly, so don't necessarily copy my work here!

So, you may be thinking that I just made a very compelling case for insurance, but don't act too quickly! We haven't gotten through all of the expenses!

The next thing to consider is how much health insurance costs. If you're lucky enough to have an employer who doesn't mind that you work on the road and will provide employee health benefits automatically deducted from your paycheck, this should be a slam dunk obvious decision. However, not all of us have those resources. Brad and I have only had access to employer-sponsored healthcare in the last year. Prior to that, we self-paid at the contracted company rate. **Prior to that**, we were both on COBRA, which is a continuation of your employer-sponsored healthcare, at 100% of the market rate, plus an administration fee.

The national average cost for an independent health plan in 2020 is around $462 per month, but that cost depends greatly on your location, age, and tobacco use. Some independent plans require a health exam as well.

So, let's use the national average to determine what your annual healthcare coverage cost would be:
$462 for an independent monthly health plan x 12 months = $5,544 for annual health insurance

Add that to your medical expenses:
$5,544 for annual health insurance + $575 for annual health expenses with insurance) = $6,119 in medical expenses with health insurance.

It's not quite as much of an obvious decision now, is it? If that hypothetical urgent care visit happens, having insurance and not having insurance is just a few hundred dollars different in annual expenses.

That being said, I also recommend looking into the options that are available to you. There are plans and subsidies available for those with minimal medical expenses that are much more affordable and can help with any unexpected and urgent expenses.

Additionally, if you have small children, I encourage you to do the math for each member of your family so you can gain a clear perspective on your healthcare needs as a family. If you or a little one takes after me and finds new and exciting ways to fall off of things, it might be worth it in the long run!

When choosing a plan, be sure to look at phrases like "copay," "deductible," "coinsurance," and "out of pocket maximum." Let's take a closer look:

1. Copay: This is a payment that you make each time you receive a specific service, whether that's a visit to a doctor or a prescription. Copays do not count towards your deductible, they come right out of your pocket and are typically paid directly to the provider (meaning, at the doctor's office or pharmacy, at the time of service).
2. Deductible: This is how much you have to pay each year before your medical plan starts paying co-insurance. Everything up to the limit of the deductible will be paid out of your pocket.

3. Coinsurance: Once you've paid your deductible, you and your insurance will split the bill for your medical services. You may see something like, "80% coinsurance after deductible." That means that your plan will pay 80% of each expense, and you'll pay 20%.
4. Out-of-Pocket Maximum: This is the most you will have to pay for your part of the coinsurance agreement. So, if you're paying 20% of each expense, those payments may eventually add up to the Out-of-Pocket Maximum. Once you've paid that amount, your plan will pay 100% of all expenses to the Lifetime Plan Maximum.

As much as I would love to teach a master class on understanding insurance plans again, I'll save that for another author or another book. In short, all of these numbers should be considered when evaluating your need for health insurance. I strongly urge anyone who is considering shopping for an individual or independent health plan to look at a document known as the "Summary Plan Description." This will help you carefully consider what is covered and how it is covered. For example, while my appointments with Dr. Smith, the general practitioner, have a very reasonable $20 copay, my appointments with Dr. Nelle, the chiropractor, are subject to the deductible and cost $40 each... unless I'm coming in for adjustments following an accident, and then those are subject to a $30 copay.

On top of that, you'll need to look at whether or not the plan has a national network of providers, meaning that you can receive medical coverage no matter where you and your van travel. Some plans offer Out-of-Network coverage at a higher deductible and lower coinsurance rate, so you'll want to be sure to visit only in-network providers whenever possible. Thankfully, it's pretty easy to research the network from each plan's customer website, or by contacting customer service.

It's enough to make the mind spin!

There's less to say about dental and vision insurance, since these types of coverages tend to be more straightforward. However, one thing to note when looking at these coverages is the plan's annual maximum, if any.

Some types of coverage do have a limit on what they'll cover in a year, so if you have a large dental emergency while on the road, you might be looking at a large bill. Additionally, most vision plans provide a free examination and an allowance on glasses or contacts, so depending on your vision needs, this may not even be worth the expense.

In conclusion, your choice to carry or not carry medical insurance really depends on whether or not it makes financial sense for your particular situation. I sincerely urge anyone to really take the time to do the math – ALL of the math – if this is a question in your mind.

## Chapter 2: Nutrition and Eating for You

Food and eating are tricky in a van. I'm not just talking about how hard it is to balance a burrito on the steering wheel while you're cruising down the highway, either. I mean that many humans are pretty domesticated when it comes to food, food storage, and cooking. When you aren't going to the grocery store regularly to fill your beautiful refrigerator and freezer with fresh ingredients, when you don't have your choice from a handful of stirring utensils, and when there's no option to plant a garden each summer, you have to become inventive.

What's the first thing you do when you're going on a road trip? For most of us, it's a stop to the gas station where we fill up the tank, and then run inside for a whole bunch of snacks! Big, sugary, caffeinated drinks to keep us awake when the road becomes monotonous, and a whole bunch of delicious junk food that we can ONLY get at gas stations quickly fill the cup holders and seats, preparing to fuel the humans in the vehicle for the adventure ahead.

When I asked around amongst my kindred van lifers about health and wellness on the road, literally the first thing everyone mentioned was reducing junk food intake. This makes sense; after all, the temptation to abandon all nutrition is incredibly high when you live on the road. There will be stretches of road where your only options for caloric intake will be found at gas stations and fast-food drive-thrus. There will be even more times when the only options for sustenance are things that can be found in your van.

Furthermore, if you have a full day of driving planned, snacking is one way to take the boredom out of long, flat stretches of road where the scenery looks the same for miles and miles. Eating not only releases endorphins, which are a nice change of pace for a stagnant brain, but also gives you something to think about besides the monotony. Staring at the scrub brush flatlands of southern Texas made me so anxious for a change of scenery that I drank an entire liter of Topo Chico to wash down a giant concha I bought at a gas station. I have no regrets about the concha - it was handmade and delicious - but I can't tell you if I was actually hungry, or just ready to occupy my senses with something other than scrub and highway heat mirages.

Personally, I think that sampling a community's cuisine is an important part of learning about the culture. I'm incredibly inspired by Anthony Bourdain, Andrew Zimmern, and Samantha Brown, and their anthropological approach to food as a huge part of a cultural experience. I would encourage anyone who is traveling in new places to try every new flavor, texture, and ingredient they can get their hands on, because food is an incredible expression of who we are as people.

That being said, our bodies aren't designed to run exclusively on high fat, high salt, high sugar diets. As my friend and fellow van dweller Katie is fond of saying, "You've got to run a vegetable through the system once in a while." Thankfully, there are more and more nutritious items that can be found easily. From packages of raw carrots and other veggies to low-fat, vegan, and gluten-free snack options that offer vitamins, fiber, and protein. Snack culture is catching up with the needs of nutrition.

Nutrition isn't just some big hoax brought to us by Big Diet Culture. The body does need a certain amount of vitamins and minerals to operate properly. From the digestive system to maintaining brain function, eating delivers the chemicals our body requires to live and thrive. The consequences of poor nutrition aren't that great, either- constipation, diarrhea, heartburn, fatigue, poor concentration, muscle weakness and dizziness... None of these symptoms are helpful for those who need to be on the road for long hours.

Therefore, eating on the road becomes a delicate balance of trying new things, while still being sure to get those fruits and veggies in, and keep regular salt, sugar, and fat intake at reasonable levels.

Another consideration in nutritional maintenance? Remembering to eat. When I lived in a house and worked in an office, the cues were always there to eat. Around noon, everyone starts heading out for lunch. Around 3pm, the afternoon doldrums creep in and it's time for a snack. After work, everyone wants dinner and bed. Radio and television commercials are specifically timed to get you thinking about your appetite. Even social media ads for food products are perfectly timed to coincide with meal times!

When you live in a van, far from the radio or the television, you don't get these prompts. Thankfully, someone had installed a CD player in our van before it came into our lives, but there was no AUX jack for streaming, no Bluetooth... in fact, not all of the speakers even worked. You don't realize how out of touch you are until you end up splurging on a hotel for the night and become absolutely entranced with commercials. Without social cues to eat, there were many days when, after morning caffeine, Brad and I would watch the sun setting on the road ahead of us and ask each other if we had eaten that day. Van life can literally be feast or famine.

Therefore, the first rules of van nutrition are as follows:
1. Experience culture through food
2. Nutrition is important
3. Remember to eat (and not always junk food!)

**The Importance of Proper Food Storage**

You might be thinking, "That's great, Kristine, but where am I getting all of these nutritious ingredients, and where am I putting them?" If there is one area in which van life is frustrating, it's definitely in the kitchen area.

If you have designed your van or skoolie with a functioning refrigerator and running water, you have made an excellent investment towards your health and wellness. In fact, when I broached the topic of food storage with other van dwellers, they literally could not fathom not having at least a refrigerator. Be it known, you do not need a refrigerator in order to be a legitimate van lifer who cares about their health and nutrition.

On our first time out, Brad and I didn't plan on having perishable goods. There was just no room for storing things that needed to be chilled, so we packed lots of high-quality low-sodium canned veggies, and whenever possible, bought local produce in small quantities that we could eat in one sitting. That, of course, brought on its own problems, because then we had to use our limited water supply to prepare veggies, and we felt incredibly guilty if we weren't able to eat it all.

We remedied this with a cooler that requires ice. Without a power supply, that was really the only option we had. And, as a bonus, the cooler could double as a seat, and the melted ice became cool, refreshing bathwater in the desert.

The problem with a cooler is that you really have to be on the beam at all times. For example, anything you place in a cooler must be in a water-tight container. Otherwise, the container will fill with water as the ice melts, and eventually, enough sloshing around will jar the contents of the container loose, filling your cooler with really wet hummus and cheese, for example. So far, the only way we have found to remove really pungent odors from a cooler is a blasting from a do-it-yourself car wash hose and a liberal application of Dawn dish soap.

Therefore, if you're going to use a cooler, I strongly recommend bringing along a full set of water-tight reusable containers, and transferring any fresh perishable food to the container immediately. By "immediately," I mean, "in the parking lot of the grocery store or market." This tends to be the easiest place to get things done because you're parked and have a place to dispose of the wrappers and original containers once you've placed everything safely in their new vessels.

The next tip for keeping a functioning cooler is to try as hard as possible to keep up with the ice levels. While having a bit of water for a bird bath is a great idea, a cooler full of tepid water is a huge temptation for bugs and smells bad. Also, most cold food is intended to remain cold, and as the temperature rises, the breeding of bad bacteria begins, creating the perfect storm of food poisoning. No one has time for this, especially if they live in a home on wheels.

I noticed that there are plenty of free-standing ice stations across the southern United States, especially in areas where fishing and hunting are very popular. These are great resources for van people, as you can generally park nearby and attend to your cooler situation in detail. Of course, most gas stations and grocery stores also sell ice, and it's relatively inexpensive.

Unfortunately, ice isn't one of those things you can just buy extra of- you can only put so much in the cooler, and then the rest melts. To offset this expense, I recommend purchasing drinking water quality ice and filling your water bottles with any excess ice that won't fit in the cooler. Excess ice can always be used somewhere. It can also be placed in spray bottles for spritz baths, saved for bathing and dishes, or incorporated into your toilet set up.

The next dilemma is keeping bugs and critters away from your food. Flies are going to be everywhere. Even if you have fantastic window screens and an amazing central air system in your van, the next time you open a door, flies, mosquitoes, and gnats are going to take advantage of the invitation to check out the inside of your awesome van. Spiders and centipedes (and worst of all- desert millipedes) will find a way in through some tiny, impossible hole somewhere. Smaller animals can slither up through the motor and make their way through the maze to the cabin. Once they're inside, the feast is on!

Your cooler and your refrigerator will typically have a seal that makes them impenetrable to insects and small animals, so we'll focus the attention of these endeavors on your dry goods. Cans are generally not a problem, either - they're not interesting. But any cardboard boxes or bags that you may have lying about are fair game.

I strongly recommend placing food items inside a tough rubber tote, particularly one that locks. These bins are smell-proof, which means they won't draw bears, coyotes, and raccoons to your van, and they are tight enough to prevent even the smallest flying creature from digging in. You can use a medium-sized tote for long term food storage, and smaller versions for your day-to-day snacks, or things you might wish to access from the front of the van.

Another great solution for storing dry food is plastic drawers. You may have built in a beautiful wooden cabinet in your van, and I commend you for doing so. However, if you store food in them, there are many small creatures in the wild with teeth that are made for gnawing through that gorgeous wooden patina. Additionally, these types of drawers and cabinets don't have the air-tight seal of a rubber bin, and insects will thrive in a bag of unattended crackers or cereal.

Anything airtight with a closing, locking lid should be sufficient. I've even seen some creative souls use large canisters and jars for storing various dry ingredients. My only caution is to make sure you have a way of securing those jars in transit, or your noggin might meet an unpleasant surprise the next time you open a cabinet or drawer.

Again, if you have the ability to transfer everything to a container that can be fully sealed, you'll be much better off. Does this take some of the spontaneity out of grocery shopping? Yes. Does this mean you have to be more mindful of your food levels? Absolutely. Will you find some food turning stale or going off before you can finish it? Unfortunately, yes, especially if you're a one or two-person van outfit.

One of the challenges of buying food for a nomadic lifestyle is that you have to be prepared to use it in many different ways. The carrots that you had for a snack earlier can be added to the stir fry you make later tonight. The lettuce from last night's salad can be the basis for today's sandwich. Whatever food products you buy, you have to be prepared to eat them right away, and until they're gone. Generally speaking, you can get two meals out of produce, one or two out of dairy products, and meat is best eaten immediately. If you have a high-powered refrigerator or freezer, these limits can be extended. Additionally, block cheese travels surprisingly well, as long as it doesn't get wet!

When you shop for food in a stationary home, you generally stock up for the week, or even the month. There are a lot of impulse purchases and ingredients bought for one specific meal or dish. In a van, even with a refrigerator, it's not quite that simple. Camper fridges are much smaller than the one you have at home, for starters, and require a significant amount of power to run appropriately. You're not going to have a bowl of fruit on the counter for folks to grab as they walk by, because that will turn into a Tim Burton-esque masterpiece of infestation very quickly. You probably won't be able to stock five different types of yogurt, and leftovers are going to be an exercise in delicacy and deliberation, between storage and reheating them. Bread can be tricky, too, as more humid areas will turn a loaf into a moldy garden almost immediately. Everything edible will need to be carefully considered before it enters the van, or your waste will quickly add up.

Based on all of this information, you may be pretty convinced that cooking a healthful meal while living in a van is pretty much impossible. Somewhere in your camping psyche, you may be stuck on traditional campfire meals, such as hot dogs diligently roasted on sticks, beans cooked in a can, and the sticky, crunchy delight of a sweet s'mores treat.

While you can absolutely indulge in what Brad and I call "The Campsite Classic" from time to time, eating hot dogs every meal, every day, for any length of time is probably appealing to only the most discerning toddler. It's also not exactly nutritionally balanced.

One of the best investments any hard-core camper, van lifer, or boondocker can make is a portable propane burner. Most versions are small, which translates to "travels well." They're easy to find at home improvement stores, hardware stores, or places that sell camping goods.

These small burners typically require an equally tiny propane tank, typically sold at the same location as the burner. While having equipment that is small in size is wonderful for stashing it in the compromised living quarters of a van, it also means that you'll only get so many meals out of each tank. Therefore, you'll likely want to have more than one on hand at all times. You'll also need to be conscious of how long it takes to make meals.

Another factor in the space vs. time vs. nutrition trifecta is your kitchenware. It may be tempting to pack up all of your cookware, especially if you're very experienced and adept in the kitchen; the truth is that you can get away with a very minimal list of supplies and still have everything you need to eat well every day.

If you've read any of my other van books, you'll know that Brad and I have compartmentalized everything that would be a "room" into a heavy-duty tote of its own. His office, which consists of a gazebo-style tent, folding table, and folding chair, along with his minimalistic approach to office supplies, takes up one tote. We have an emergency tote, which includes jumper cables, a tire changing kit, road flares, first aid kits (yes, plural. We'll talk about those in a minute), tarp, bungee cable tie-downs, funnels, a tool kit, and related mechanical supplies in another tote. Our bed linens have their own smaller tote, while the laundry has a bag within a tote.

The kitchen, therefore, has its own tote, which is surprisingly smaller than you would imagine. Our burner actually came in its own housing, so it lives on its own behind the driver's seat. The propane tanks are in the tote, along with the following:

- One 3-quart pot
- A cast iron skillet
- Three forks, three spoons, two steak knives
- One multi-function can opener
- One spatula and one non-slotted cooking spoon
- Two large plates
- Two large bowls
- Two each dish rags and dish towels
- One dishpan
- One small bottle of environmentally friendly dish soap

The rest of the room in this particular tote is devoted to canned and dry goods for several reasons. First, canned soup, tuna, pasta, peanut butter, beans, and instant rice are all great staples to have on-hand for an actual rainy day. They heat up quickly without draining the propane, and with little mess or fuss. Second, refer back to the part where we keep our dry goods locked up to prevent infestation. Cans aren't in as much danger, obviously, but keeping everything centralized makes it so much easier. Lastly, the weight of the cans prevents the tote from shifting too much while we drive. That means we can strategically stack it next to a lighter or currently empty tote to prevent things from slamming around in the back as we drive over treacherous terrain.

Depending on how many people live in your van, you may want more or less in your kitchen set up. If you have a gorgeous skoolie, you might not need a tote at all as you'll have significantly more room for cabinets, drawers, and other storage spaces. I simply provide this information as a guide to how little you can truly get away with packing while still being able to create delicious, healthy meals.

**Cooking for Your Crowd**

In the References section, I've included several links to recipe sources to help you get an idea of the types of meals you can make with just one burner, one pot, and one pan. Sure, it requires a little creativity, but you'll eventually get the hang of it. My cooking style when we first hit the road was "slop everything in a pot and make it taste good." This meant a lot of stews, stir frys, chilis, fajitas, and pasta with all of the veggies we needed to use up quickly thrown in. Honestly, it wasn't a bad strategy, given the "two meal" rule I mentioned earlier for fresh produce. That being said, there came a time when I felt like we were just eating slop after slop.

One of the most enjoyable parts of traveling the country is experiencing the local cuisine, as I mentioned earlier. But you don't have to do that exclusively at a restaurant. In Louisiana, for example, we stopped by a local market and picked up some amazing alligator sausages, which we grilled at a campsite and served over rice and veggies made with a local dry spice blend. We finished up the meal with a two-person pecan pie that we picked up at a bakery just a mile away from the campsite entrance. In Seattle, we feasted on a meal plucked directly from Pike Place Market, including cheese from Beecher's, salmon from Totem's Smokehouse, along with cherries and an avocado we picked up as we were strolling through the colorful stalls and aisles of the busy market. No cooking was required, and I'll always fondly remember that meal. We found an out-of-season camping spot by a lake several dozen miles away, and after a quick swim, we ate our feast out of the paper bags they came in while we watched the sunset, tired and dripping wet.

That being said, it's a little easier to cook for two unwavering foodies. If your diet, palette, or family include special requirements, you're obviously going to need to keep those at the forefront of your meal planning.

If anyone in your caravan has allergies, I strongly recommend eliminating ingredients that would cause an allergic reaction, simply because cross-contamination in tight quarters is extremely likely. This is, of course, ultimately up to you and your traveling companions, but my experiences with trying to keep a van clean (which we'll get to shortly, as well) have me erring on the side of caution.

If you are a parent who finds themselves cooking multiple meals for multiple picky children (or even grown family members) at home, you might want to find a way to streamline this experience on the road. For example, on stir fry night, let everyone choose their own veggies from the existing supply, and cook each plate individually. No substitutions, no replacements. Run your outdoor kitchen like a fast-paced diner! If someone doesn't want to participate in campfire chili, let them choose from one of the rainy day canned options, or perhaps enjoy a campfire quesadilla. While bread, buns, and rolls succumb easily to the elements, tortillas, naan, and pita tend to hold up well when the weather changes rapidly. Plus, if you're intrepid enough, you can make your own tortillas or naan with your cast iron skillet! Allowing for some variation on the menu isn't a problem, but cooking several different meals with one pot or pan and one burner will become time-consuming and frustrating very quickly. I know many van parents who have ended up having instant oatmeal and protein bars for dinner now and again just to create a compromise before bedtime!

## A Drop About Hydration

One thing that is often forgotten in the context of van life is staying hydrated. When we're thirsty at home or in an office, we walk to the sink, water fountain, or water filter to pour a glass of water, drink it, and move on with our lives. In a van scenario, you may not have running water, or you may only have grey water. You'll also want to pay attention to the side effects of constant hydration, as well. You may not have a toilet in your van, which means you'll need to find public restroom stops as you travel or make like the bears and use the woods. I have to agree, all of this is a hassle.

At the same time, the side effects of dehydration aren't that pleasant, either. Headaches, muscle cramps, dizziness, and fatigue will put a real damper on your van adventure. You do need to drink plenty of water to keep your organs functioning and your mind alert.

One easy way to do this is to fill up on clean water every chance you get. Nearly every National Park has a free water station, where you can fill up your personal water bottles, or even reuse gallon jugs with fresh water for the next leg of your journey. If you're lucky enough to visit Hot Springs, there are spring water filling stations as well so you can take the famed healing waters on the road with you.

Reusable water bottles are ideal, but they do require cleaning and occasionally become damaged or leak. Don't take that as an opportunity to ignore hydration! Keep up with the cleanliness, and use disposable bottles as necessary to keep you healthy in the meantime. You can always drop them off at a recycling center later.

As you're enjoying the new flavors and snacks found around the country, look at beverage options as well. There are lots of interesting regional juices and sodas that deserve exploration. It's true that high amounts of sugar and caffeine aren't exactly great for your body, but as always, moderation is key.

The same can be said of alcohol, with an added note that you should never operate a van or skoolie under the influence. Brad and I are craft beer fans who visited many breweries on the first leg of our journey, and nearly every bartender checked in to make sure we were good before we tried to leave. It is much better to hang out in a parking lot for a few extra hours than to drive while buzzed. Instead, consider getting cans, bottles, or growlers to go, putting them in your cooler, and enjoying them after you've parked.

The last words of wisdom I'll offer when it comes to hydration are to always overstock on liquids. Weather can change quickly, and a rainy day can become a scorcher in what feels like an instant. There have been several times when Brad and I have thought we didn't need to pack water for a day of activities because the morning was cool, or the hike was short, or it was just a few miles to the next town. We deeply regretted that decision each and every time. Dehydration can be extremely dangerous, and affect you quickly, especially when you're outside, so err on the side of caution!

The temptation to snack more, to eat at restaurants more frequently, and to abandon everything we've learned about nutrition is very high when on the road. Without access to a full kitchen with adequate refrigeration, a large freezer, running water, and all the gadgets and gizmos that make meal prep so simple, you may feel a bit lost and overwhelmed. Take the time to browse recipes for new ideas. Spend some time at local markets to give each meal a unique flare. Consider multiple uses for each ingredient you buy. Most of all, be very mindful of food storage to ensure you aren't inviting bugs, critters, mold, or other contaminants into the van!

## Chapter 3: Exercise: "Moving More Than a Van"

If one were to create a Venn diagram of people who love being outdoors and those who love van life, the overlap would be significant, if not a near-complete eclipse. It makes sense, of course. If you don't care for tall trees, a nice breeze, and the steady drone of mosquitos, you probably ought to choose a less untamed type of home.

In fact, many of the people who have chosen van life do so because of the proximity to nature and the ability to experience so much of the beauty and wilderness that is still abundant on this planet. That means ample opportunities to hike, climb, canoe, bike, and participate in all of the amazing outdoor sports and activities that bring us closer to peace and harmony with Earth itself.

All of this outdoor adventuring requires a lot of energy, and many van nomads log hundreds - if not thousands - of miles outside of the van. But there's one fact that is often overlooked; you have to drive hundreds - if not thousands - of miles to get from place to place. The unfortunate truth is that some days will be dedicated to sunrise to sunset driving, with no hiking, no biking, and little activity besides getting out of the van, filling up with gas, and getting back into the van.

Additionally, not every day is going to be perfect for outdoor activities. Rock climbing in a lightning storm is a pretty bad idea. Canoeing on ice requires specialized equipment. There are days when even taking a little walk around your campsite may seem like a major and unnecessary undertaking, either because of your physical status, your mental or emotional state, or just plain gross weather. If you're working from the road, you may find it occasionally difficult to fit in those all-day hikes when you have meetings or looming deadlines as well.

All of these factors compound the importance of maintaining physical fitness while living in a van. The good news is that there are several things you can do to keep yourself feeling great and ready to take on spontaneous adventures, even when the weather, your travel plans, or your mind and body don't want to cooperate.

**A few things before we get started:**

1. Don't do any type of exercise that doesn't feel good. Everyone has some kind of limitation, so don't push yourself beyond what you can comfortably do today. Just because you saw someone else do it on social media, because you feel like you ought to be able to do it, or because I mentioned it here in this book, doesn't mean you should rush out to bend yourself into a specific routine.

    In my case, I spent my teenage years and early twenties working with rescue horses. As a result, I have a lot of unpredictable limitations in my body. Combine that with the fact that I am clumsy enough to break and sprain things just walking across a room, and you're probably wincing as hard as all of the physical therapists I've worked with over the years. I creak. I don't bend correctly. And that's totally okay, because that's just how my body is.
    So, the number one rule is to work with your body. Don't force it. Push yourself, but not into the danger zone. Listen to your joints and muscles. Listen to your medical support team. Most importantly, if climbing mountains makes you want to punch a tree (guilty) don't do it!

2. Don't feel like you need to do anything just because #vanlife stars on social media do it. The first major disappointment I had about living in a van was that it is not pretty. There are tons of pictures online of gorgeous, perfectly toned young men and women with perfect skin and hair, in their gleaming white vans, wearing stylish bathing suits, romping around with their equally beautiful children, or staring peacefully at the sun setting over a picturesque beach.

When I look back at the pictures from our first year living in a van, I feel like I can smell Brad and myself through the photographs. There will be dirt, mud, sand, and bugs. There will be stink. In fact, there will be all kinds of stink from all sorts of sources while you figure out your own process. You will have to go to the bathroom in the wilderness at some point, and you may not be graceful. You will probably run out of water at some point and have to deal with sticky, sand-filled hair. You will sweat from places you didn't know could produce sweat.

So, let's go ahead and abandon that perfect social media picture, okay? Swerving back into reality, not every van lifer hikes, bikes, or climbs. I've heard whispers that you're not really a van person until you've done Angel's Landing, or you're not a hiker if you haven't done the Grand Canyon. That's all bunk. If you want to do Angel's Landing, go for it. Be safe. Send me pictures. Everyone experiences the planet in different ways that are meaningful and enjoyable for them. Don't make yourself miserable because you think you need to do something, and don't be hard on yourself if these goals are not accessible to you.

Here's my true-life example: Brad and I did the Mighty Five in Utah in May of 2018. To the uninitiated, that's Arches, Canyonlands, Capitol Reef, Bryce Canyon, and Zion national parks, back-to-back. We started with Canyonlands, and my inner mountain goat was having a blast, hopping from rock to rock, following mysteriously placed cairns across the tops of wind-swept plateaus. And then, because I'm me, I misjudged a foot-wide hop from one rocky outcrop to another, and slid in between the rocks, twisting my ankle on the way. At the time, it was no big deal - I walked it out, finished the hike, and loved every minute of it.

The next day at Capitol Reef, I found the going pretty tough. At Arches, I was pretty much dragging my swollen foot. Then, I made the critical error of green-lighting the Navajo-Peekaboo Trail at Bryce Canyon, which is approximately five miles in length with nearly 1,500-foot elevation gain, and I fell apart. By the time we got to Zion, I couldn't tell you which hurt more, my ankle or my pride.

So, the moral of the story is that there is no such thing as the perfect social media-washed #vanlifer. Pushing past that point of comfort, fitness, and desire will only end in tears and the need for medical treatment.

With that advice in hand, let's take a look at some of the types of exercise that are conducive to van living. We'll focus on how to stay in shape while you're actively on the road and helpful tips for finding fitness outlets when you feel like mixing it up a bit.

**Regular Activity for Those Who Wander**
Hiking, biking, climbing, and paddling aren't the only activities available to those who live in a van. It is perfectly okay to go for the occasional walk to wander around, get fresh air, and explore the scenery. While hiking often includes long trails, varied landscape, and obstacles of different levels of difficulty, you can pause for a minute to take a slow, easy, and pointless walk. Look at the different types of trees. Focus on your surroundings more than logging the miles.

If speed is more your thing, go for a jog! There are plenty of trails around the country that are absolutely beautiful and manicured for joggers and runners to take advantage of. Many national parks offer horseback riding trails, which are a great workout for the core and legs, and an amazing way to experience the gorgeous settings. Go for a swim, or rent an inner tube and do a float/hike combination down a nearby waterway. Don't feel you have to do the same thing over and over!

There are plenty of exercises that translate well to the outdoor experience which might surprise you. Doing Yin Yoga on the beach in Hawaii opened up my eyes to the fact that I didn't need a studio with a guru giving me directions in order to enjoy my practice. In fact, I found that breaking up a long hike with a few intervals of yoga poses, such as a quick Sun Salutation, or a Warrior/Sun flow, helped me avoid stiffness in my lower back and hamstrings. If you're not interested in doing chaturangas in the dirt, don't worry about bringing your mat, a softer spot with no rocks or branches, and a towel should do the trick!

Speaking of intervals, you can also incorporate high intensity interval training (HIIT) moves into your van life as well. HIIT workouts may seem impossible outside of the gym, but Tabata circuits of burpees, squats, lunges, mountain climbers, and planks are all bodyweight exercises that can be done absolutely anywhere. As an added bonus, no one will be around to hear you curse while you do burpees.

**"Extended Driving Pose" Is Not An Exercise**
What about those days during which you spend more time seated behind the wheel than you do standing or moving? If you've ever driven twelve hours straight, you are aware of the physical and mental strain it can put on a person. First, your behind goes completely numb. Then, your legs start to hurt and your shoulders get tense from holding onto the wheel. If you drive an elderly vehicle with a sense of humor, your fingers probably get a little numb and tingly from trying to accommodate for the lack of power steering. Your lumbar region starts to feel like a jigsaw puzzle put together incorrectly. Your head hurts, none of your music is worth listening to, and you start to dream of a heating pad, a massage, and one of those astronaut beds they advertise on late night infomercials.

If you've never driven twelve hours straight, don't let this description dissuade you from trying. The key to keeping the body happy during long hauls is movement. While there are very few exercises you can actually do behind the wheel, this is a good time to take advantage of the notoriously low fuel economy of your van or skoolie, and move every time you stop for gas.

When I say "move," I mean really move. Not the casual "nobody's watching, right?" micro stretches you can do while pumping your gas or scraping insect carcasses off of your vehicle's front end. I mean, really go for it and get the blood flowing again.

There are several ways you can do this. My recommendation would be to incorporate at least one exercise from each section of this chart before you hop back into the van again. If you're bold, do them right there in the parking lot. If you're less enthusiastic about making a scene in your travel clothes with car seat hair, try sneaking into the back of your vehicle or the restroom - the walk will do you good!

| Basic Stretches | Road Yoga | Cardio |
| --- | --- | --- |
| • Bend over and touch your toes | • Mountain pose to forward fold, halfway lift, back to mountain pose | • Walk rapidly in place while you pump your gas (yes, people will look at you strangely, but your legs and spine will LOVE it) |
| • Reach all the way to the sky | • Warrior 1 and Reverse Warrior (Peaceful Warrior) | |
| • Stand on your tippy-toes, then relax through your heels (best done on a curb so you can stretch all the way through!) | • Side Angle/ Extended Side Angle Pose (or variations) | • Jumping jacks |
| | | • High knees |
| | • Chair pose | • Goblet squats (substitute a water bottle for a kettlebell) |
| • Reach your arm down the side of your leg to the ground | • Low lunge to Runner's Lunge | |
| | • Supine Twists (you may want to do these in the back of your van) | • Jog around the parking lot for a few minutes |
| • Slow long lunges | | • Use a curb or sidewalk for a few minutes of step ups |
| • Stand with legs hip-width apart and touch the opposite hand to opposite toes | • Downward Facing Dog (again, you probably don't want to put your hands on the parking lot or bathroom floor) | • Squat jumps |
| | | • Incline push ups against the van |
| • Chest openers | | |
| • Small circles and big circles in both directions (do this with your head, your arms, your hands, and your ankles for a full-body release!) | • Extended triangle pose | |

These are just a few examples, of course. Your body will tell you exactly what type of motion is going to feel best when you get out of the driver's seat. Speaking of which, I'd like to caution you to always exit your van slowly, and pay attention to where your feet might be landing. I can't tell you how many times Brad and I have managed to fall out of the driver's seat because we underestimated how rubbery and unsteady our legs were after a long stretch of driving. Additionally, take your time when fully standing up. Orthostatic hypotension (drops in your blood pressure) is a very real thing, and if you think doing jumping jacks at a gas pump is too embarrassing, you'll definitely not want to faint at one! Take your time swinging in and out of your vehicle to avoid any injury or awkwardness.

**Outside of the Outdoors**

There may also be times when you crave indoor fitness. If you're a very outdoorsy person, this may not make sense right off the bat, but there are many reasons why you might find yourself longing for the gym or a workout class.

The first is air conditioning. A controlled, indoor environment is going to provide a lot of advantages for those who are trying to "level up" with their outdoor activities. There are many scales available that rate various hikes, climbs, and summits as different grades or classes, based on how difficult they are to complete. As you "climb" the ranks (pun mostly intended), you'll need to gain certain physical attributes and abilities in order to be successful. If your van or skoolie is not the right environment for building those upper body muscles, or gaining strength in your legs, you may wish to check out a gym or fitness group to boost your workouts.

You may also just want a change of pace. I discovered in my early 20s that a boxing class here and there is wonderful for relieving my anxiety and frustration. Since there are few things in nature that tolerate jabs, punches, and kicks quite like a punching bag, the most ideal outlet for this type of release is a dedicated boxing gym.

Lastly, you might just want the company. We'll talk about all of the interesting things van life can do to your mental health in a bit, but many of us are hardwired to really enjoy exercising in groups. Whether that means taking an aerobics class or Aqua Zumba or swinging from a TRX strap, you may find a great deal of enjoyment in working out with others. There's camaraderie and a touch of competition. Best of all, you're not suffering alone.

When these urges appear, go ahead and indulge them, if you're financially capable of doing so at that moment. Many gyms or studios have a "drop in" policy that you can easily find on their website or by giving them a quick call. For a reduced rate, you can usually appear once, take advantage of the equipment or teacher's knowledge, enjoy your workout, enjoy the showers with endless hot water, and be on your way. Always check it out ahead of time, though, so you know when to arrive, and abide by any dress codes or other policies. Some studios or gyms require specific footwear, for example, or ask that drop-ins only come during specific non-peak hours. Usually these notes are posted on the website, so you aren't taken by surprise.

Another option is to find a gym or club with national access. This is a relatively new phenomenon, but there are many chain gyms that allow members to use any of their locations across the United States. Again, I recommend double-checking policies ahead of time to be adequately prepared, but there is something very convenient about being able to stop by a completely new-to-you gym in a state you've never visited before and knocking out a few miles on the treadmill before hopping back in your van and heading out again. And yes, included-with-membership showers and massage chairs are a fantastic added bonus.

You can also take advantage of municipal Health Trails. The actual name used will depend on your location, of course, but the concept is the same. Along a few miles of walking, biking, or hiking trails, there will be a variety of obstacles or fitness challenges set up. The instructions are posted so you know how to properly execute the exercise, along with a recommended number of reps or time allotted to complete the practice. Often, the equipment can be multi-purposed for several different exercises, such as balance beams that can be used for step ups, or a bar that can be used for pull-ups or knee raises.

Locating these types of trails may seem like a daunting challenge, since they go by many different names, but I suggest starting with a search for "trails near me," and refining from there. Terms like "fitness," "wellness," and "challenge" are frequent indicators that a trail features some additional obstacles to help you add variety to your overall workout routine.

Again, it's important to note that you should not feel obligated to do anything that is uncomfortable, unrealistic, or potentially dangerous. Always stretch before and after you exercise. When going on long adventures, be sure to pack plenty of water and snacks to fuel your body, particularly snacks that are high in protein and energy. Be mindful of your body's warning signs, and if you feel discomfort approaching, find a way to safely end the activity and return to the van as quickly as possible.

This section may seem like a bunch of obvious reminders. Go to the doctor. Brush your teeth. Eat your vegetables. Get some exercise. At the heart of it, yes, those are all things many of us learned in elementary school, if not before. Nevertheless, there's something magical that happens any time we make huge changes in our lives that often causes us to abandon some of the things we know we ought to do as we adapt to our new method of survival.

If you find yourself six months into your van quest, and you haven't yet seen a dentist, do not despair. This doesn't mean you're an unhealthy or neglectful person. You've obviously had much bigger things on your mind, like where to go next, finding a place to sleep and rest every night, how to deal with road problems, possible van breakdowns, and more. Forgive yourself and make it up to yourself in the near future.

The same goes for eating healthfully and getting enough exercise. If you find that you're not where you want to be, give yourself some grace, set new goals, and act more conscientiously. I know that's easier said than done, especially if you have mile after mile of endless driving to rehash all of your mistakes.

But let's be honest – adapting to van life is hard. It's like moving into a new apartment every single day for the first several months. You have no idea where anything is. You're not sure if the furniture is in the right place. It is possible to run out of water, and sometimes you don't have enough power to charge your phone. Unusual problems will arise. You're trying to build routines when very little is the same from day to day. You're allowed to have a few hiccups in practical living.

Hopefully, the reminders in this book will help you either stay on the path of preventive care, or at least make it easier to navigate back to a regular wellness outlook if you find yourself straying. If you haven't started your voyage yet, I hope that you're able to use these points and reminders as a jumping-off place for integrating the basic preventive care you practice at home into your less domesticated van lifestyle. At the very least, you'll have a new collection of tricks, tips, and van life hacks that you can incorporate into your next adventure!

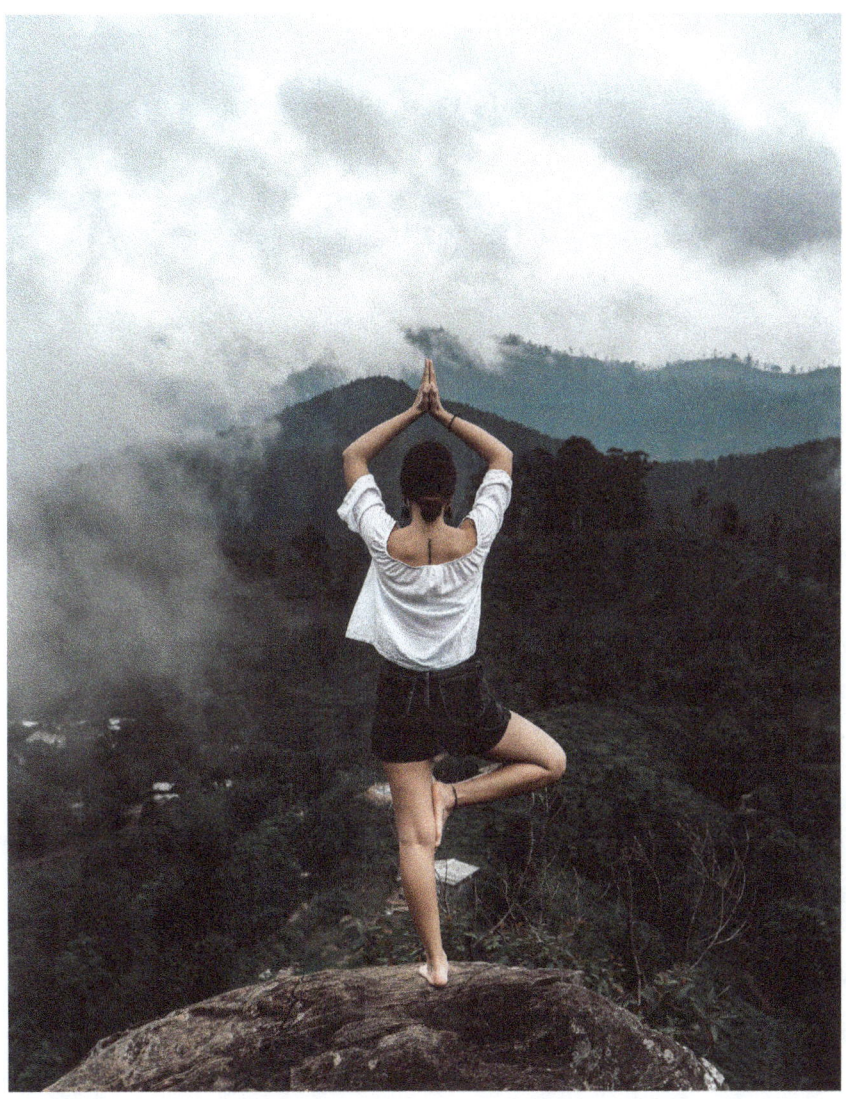

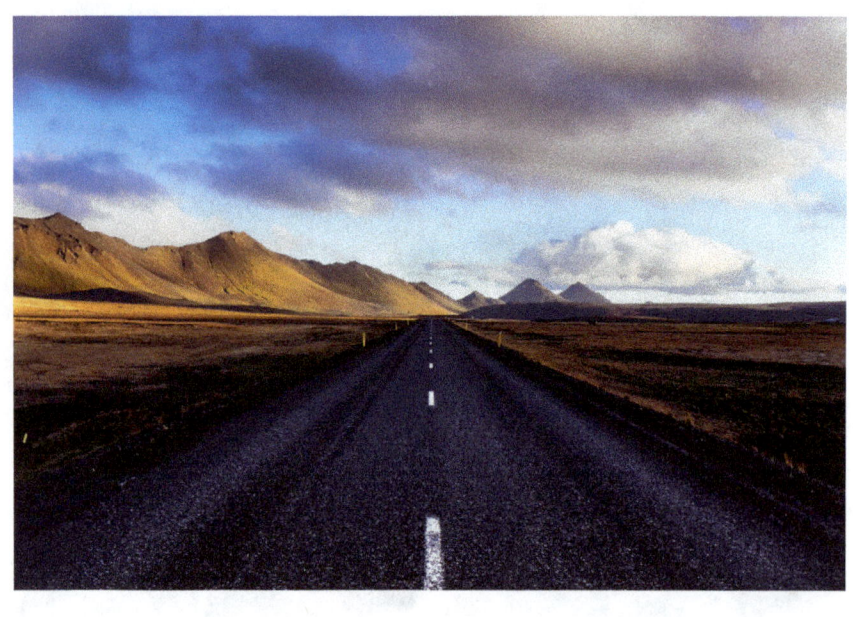

# Section 3: Managing Less Than Perfect Health on the Road

I'd love to tell you that if you do everything exactly right from the last section, that you'll always be healthy and happy. Unfortunately, the human body doesn't work like that. You can see every doctor you need on a regular basis, wash your hands copiously, eat the largest quantities of the freshest vegetables possible, hydrate to perfection, and still fall prey to illness or injury.

When we get sick or injured while living in a house, condo, or apartment, the solution is obvious; we climb into bed or make a nest on the sofa, and rest in between watching daytime television, nibbling on crackers, sipping ginger ale, and downing our preferred medications. We have ice packs and heating pads and plenty of pillows to pad our sick beds, and it's generally just a short, wobbly trip to the bathroom.

On the road, all of that is turned on its head. Of course, you can turn your sleeping area into a nest for recuperation, and if your van or skoolie has a bathroom, it's going to be closer than ever. But there are also many less convenient aspects to being sick or injured in a van. You have to decide whether to push on, or stay put. You need to find places to rest more frequently. You have to be more concerned about spreading germs. If you're injured, even getting in and out of the van can become tricky.

My number one recommendation is to be as prepared as possible for illnesses and injuries. In this section, we'll take a look at dealing with both chronic conditions and emergency situations in the context of van life. During our first year on the road, I think Brad and I managed to experience the worst bout of health-related situations we'd had in years, so a lot of the information I'll present is based on my own anecdotes. However, everyone on the road has issues at some point. So, I've pulled in a lot of thoughts and recommendations from experts in healthcare and vanlife, and sometimes both. These tips help guide us all through what are often the worst days of our van journey.

**Disclaimer: This Book Is Not a Doctor**

One quick disclaimer before we proceed: Always follow your physician's advice when it comes to your medical care. The following tips are not intended to replace any recommendations from healthcare professionals. While you are ultimately in charge of your own wellness, please consider the guidelines shared with you by actual, trained medical staff over anything I suggest. I don't know the ins and outs of your life, your health status, or your abilities. I'm just a van lifer who learned things the hard way sharing what I learned with other van lifers, so they don't have to learn it the hard way!

## Chapter 1: Managing Chronic Conditions from Anywhere and Everywhere

We touched a bit on dealing with maintenance medication and chronic conditions in the previous section, but I wanted to dive a little deeper into what it means to live on the road with a condition that won't just simply clear up on its own one day.

There's a lot of undue stigma about those who suffer from chronic conditions. The prevalent opinion is that, if people take good care of themselves through preventive care, they will not experience chronic conditions later in life. While there's some validity to that claim, many chronic conditions are based less on lifestyle choices and more on genetics, environmental factors, or sheer chance.

The term "chronic condition" refers to any health condition that persists for longer than three months and includes:
- Alcohol Use Disorder
- Alzheimer's Disease and Related Dementia Arthritis (Osteoarthritis and Rheumatoid)
- Asthma
- Atrial Fibrillation
- Autism Spectrum Disorders
- Cancer (Breast, Colorectal, Lung, Prostate, etc.)
- Chronic Kidney Disease
- Chronic Obstructive Pulmonary Disease (COPD)

- Crohn's Disease
- Cystic Fibrosis
- Depression
- Diabetes
- Epilepsy
- Heart Failure
- Hepatitis B & C
- HIV/AIDS
- Hyperlipidemia (High cholesterol)
- Hypertension (High blood pressure)
- Ischemic Heart Disease
- Multiple Sclerosis
- Osteoporosis
- Parkinson's Disease
- Schizophrenia and Other Mental Illnesses
- Stroke
- Substance Use Disorders

I have both good news and bad news. Bad news first: Generally speaking, living in a van will not make your chronic condition go away. Here's the good news, though. Living in a van is still very much a possibility for many people coping with chronic conditions. There are certain lifestyle changes associated with van living, such as reduced stress, less air pollution, and increased physical activity, that can have a positive impact on some of the symptoms of certain chronic conditions.

That doesn't mean it will be a walk in the park. I was diagnosed with a chronic condition in 2008. So far, things have been well maintained with medication, regular check-ins with my medical support team, and even therapy as needed to help me through the rough spots. There are good days and bad days. I have been hospitalized due to complications from my condition, and I learned how to be more aware of what causes difficulties and what warning signs to look for.

Therefore, I will always recommend that anyone living with chronic conditions make their well-being a priority to prevent larger complications in the long-run.

**Be Open With Your Care Team**
The first thing I encourage anyone with a persistent medical situation to do is speak to their medical care team about their plans to live on the road.

When I first broached the subject with my primary care provider, I was expecting her to tell me she had never heard such a horrible idea. She did not. In fact, she told me she was jealous, started telling me about all sorts of cool places I needed to check out, and gave me a few pointers for starting my blog. Then, we got into the 'Real Talk' portion of the appointment where we discussed how to get my medications, how to store them properly, and what to do if I miss a dose on the road. We then scheduled our next follow-up appointment as a video conference, along with a few resources I could tap into if things started to slide sideways while I was on the road.

Most importantly, she reminded me of something I hadn't considered: It's okay to take care of yourself. By this, she meant that if I have to put a pause on van life, circle back home more frequently, or in any manner stop adventuring because I needed to prioritize myself, it's not some huge failure. It's hitting the proverbial pause button before you're forced to hit full stop and eject.

I've mentioned the #vanlife ego a few times, and I'll mention it again. There seems to be this odd social pressure to drop out of society and succeed, but if you need to make van life a part-time thing, a small radius thing, or take a break and check into a hotel for a while, it does not make you any less of a van lifer. It doesn't mean you've failed in any shape or form.

If you are currently receiving treatment for a chronic illness, by all means, you can still explore the world, as long as you have the green light from your medical team. Perhaps that means you don't sell your home and go off the grid right away, but instead, you explore a smaller radius around your home base while treatment is ongoing. Maybe that means being a "weekend warrior" for a period of time.

Once you've got the official "go ahead" from your medical team, determine if virtual check-ins are a good idea for you and where you are in treatment. Since the COVID-19 pandemic, many physicians have adapted to video conferencing for check-ins or non-emergency appointments in which labs (such as bloodwork, urinalysis, or other samples) are not required. If this is an option for you, be sure to position your van so that at the time of your appointments, you are in a secure, quiet, well-lit area with a strong WiFi signal. Make sure that the phone or laptop you'll be using has enough charge to make it through the appointment. Another kind reminder is to make sure you're taking the time zones into account. Since van lifers are notorious for losing track of what day it is, be sure to set a reminder on your phone so you don't miss your check-in entirely.

**Medication Tips**
Medications can be tricky on the road, as mentioned earlier. While using national chain pharmacies can help with obtaining your prescriptions, there are many types of prescriptions that require frequent updates from your physician to measure its effectiveness and any potentially harmful side effects. Make sure you talk to your team about your van plans so that you can adequately schedule both your appointments and travel. Missing an appointment - and thus a refill - can be incredibly harmful to your continued well-being, so make sure you stay on top of your schedule. Additionally, if you're going to miss an appointment due to unforeseen events, such as a van breakdown, bad weather, or other delays, talk to your provider as soon as possible. You don't want to wait longer than you need to for that appointment and subsequent refill.

Storing prescriptions can also be difficult. If you have prescriptions that are temperature sensitive, I recommend not taking your chances with low-tech options like a cooler. There are several tiny refrigerators on the market that can plug into your dash and won't drain your battery. By "tiny," I mean, they can fit a few cans of soda. These are often the perfect size for medications, as they can be stashed in the front of the van without the chance of tumbling around in the back. Check out your local supermarket or department store to see what options they have.

This may seem like a strange dictive, but I also recommend storing your medication in a way that you'll be able to remember whether or not you've taken them. For example, those day-of-the-week pill organizers can be incredibly helpful. When you're on the road, days tend to blur into each other and your medication routine may feel a bit disrupted.

Years ago, I trained our dog to beg for a treat every time I needed to take my medications, and as a result, I could never forget. Our old beagle would start notifying me that 'Treat Time' was coming up about fifteen minutes before I needed to take my pills. Pretty soon, I had trained my own internal clock to start anticipating this daily interruption.

On the road, however, time starts to lose meaning. You wake up when you wake up, and you go to bed when you go to bed. Aside from any potential client meetings or deadlines, days and hours seem meaningless. Your internal clock has basically given up, and there's little sense of routine. I've actually got a little two-sided sign that I flip to remind myself of medication status. One side says, "You're Good." The other says "Take Your Meds, Dear." I flip the sign to "You're Good" after I take my meds each morning, and flip it to "Take Your Meds, Dear" before I go to bed for the night. Is there plenty of room for human error? Absolutely! Yet so far, I've been pretty good about keeping track of where I am on my schedule, and hopefully you'll be inspired to create a system of alarms, alerts, or signs that work for you.

In a nutshell, managing a chronic condition from the road is entirely possible. You may have to make adjustments to your travel schedule or include certain accommodations to your overall plan, but unless your medical team specifically forbids it, there's a version of van life that is accessible to nearly everyone. Whether you have to temporarily scale back, or make very deliberate and thoughtful plans for your daily endeavors, you can find a way to incorporate van life into your lifestyle.

## Chapter 2: When Bad Things Happen

Regardless of your best efforts, you will find yourself under the weather at some point. It is my greatest hope that your van life be blessed with the best health at all times. However, the truth is that we all come down with a bug here or there, or find an exciting way to accidentally damage ourselves through the course of daily activities. Perhaps that's just my own clumsy experience, but in any lifestyle with increased activity, the chances of experiencing minor sprains and strains greatly multiply.

**Preparing for Minor Disasters**

As I mentioned in the beginning of this chapter, being prepared is key. The literal last thing you want to do when you're ill or injured is drag yourself to the pharmacy and fill your cart with a bunch of things that may or may not make you feel better. That's unnecessary exposure to the outside world, and you'll probably end up impulse buying supplies you don't really need, simply because you're desperate to feel better.

Instead, create a Medical Preparation Kit before you kick off your van life. Since real estate is at a premium inside the van, the contents of this kit should focus on things that are likely to happen to you and your family, along with some vital "just in case" type elements. In my opinion, the Med Prep Kit is more important than extra undergarments if that helps emphasize how crucial it is to really plan this part out!

You'll definitely want to include at least a basic first aid kit in your MPK. I don't just mean a multi-pack of adhesive bandages and a tube of antiseptic ointment, either. I mean an **actual first aid kit** that includes things like:

- Gauze dressing pads of various sizes (at least large and small sizes)
- Trauma pads
- Gauze roll bandages
- First aid tape roll
- Instant cold compress

- A basic triangular sling
- Adhesive bandages in every size imaginable, including Elbow/Knee patch size (2"x4"), junior size (⅜" x 1 ½ "), fingertip and knuckle type, and 1" and ¾" sizes
- Thermometer
- Triple antibiotic ointment
- Antiseptic cleaning wipes
- Hydrocortisone cream
- Aloe/Multipurpose burn cream
- Tweezers
- Scissors
- Coban-style self-adhesive wrap
- Extra clean towels
- Paper towels
- Box of disposable facial tissues (at least one)
- Duct tape

These types of first aid kits can be found at many retailers already packaged in an easy-store waterproof container and usually have a handy first aid guidebook tucked inside. Of course, you can easily build your own using this as a shopping list. I would definitely recommend making sure you have a waterproof, airtight bag or box to store these items in, and definitely spring for the guidebook as well. You may think that first aid is pretty intuitive - or at least easily Googled - until you find yourself deep in the Ozarks with no phone service, wondering how panicked you should get about a mysterious rash.

But don't stop there! There are a lot of situations that need more than bandages and a book! As my aunties recommended, having naproxen, acetaminophen, AND ibuprofen on hand isn't a bad idea. In addition, bear in mind that you don't have to purchase giant economy-sized bottles of each, unless you already go through that much at home. A small bottle will be enough to get you through the early stages of any minor ailment, and can be replenished as necessary.

If you're an allergy sufferer (as many of us are), you may want to speak to your physician about your allergy situation and come up with a backup plan, especially if this is your first time travelling extensively out of state. Your body is about to encounter brand new pollen and spores and all sorts of allergy triggers that it may never have experienced before. Depending on your current triggers and allergic responses, you might need a backup medication or epinephrine injectable on hand to prevent an unforeseen emergency. A bottle of saline nasal flush may also be something you want to keep on hand to reduce allergic responses. If your allergies can trigger an asthma attack, make sure you have emergency inhalers at the ready in your Med Prep Kit as well.

Then there's what I call the "multipurpose solution." This includes items that can assist with a variety of conditions. For example, menthol cough drops can soothe an irritated throat or cough, provide relief to an upset stomach (but can irritate heartburn symptoms, so be careful there), and even quell anxiety by encouraging deep, meaningful breathing. A menthol chest rub can also feel very nice on sore muscles and feet. A bottle of non-talc powder with calamine can be extremely helpful when dealing with chafing, burning, rashes, insect bites and stings, and help you feel less gross when it's been a long stretch between bathing opportunities.

I also recommend having a few over-the-counter remedies on hand in case something pops up. This includes a bismuth subsalicylate, like Pepto-Bismol, or similar product that can stave off upset stomachs and diarrhea. Both a daytime multi-symptom formula, and a nighttime multi-symptom formula for cold and flu are a good investment. Head colds are common anytime and anywhere, and being in a moving vehicle while you're feeling stuffy and snotty is just very uncomfortable.

Brad and I picked up some kind of bug just before we hit Virginia. I was going through a box of tissues a day by myself, and I could tell that Brad was just miserable. I had long been looking forward to doing an overnight hike at Shenandoah National Park, but what really happened is that Brad parked the van at a beautiful overlook so we could take a nap in the back. We ended up having to stop every few hours for a rest period. We pulled the daytime liquid from the Med Prep Kit and made a lot of hot tea with honey on our propane burner to help our aching heads, throats, and sinuses.

In the first year of van life, I would say we used everything in our Med Prep Kit except the adhesive bandages. I ended up using a lot of Coban and gauze wrap for my assorted sprains and strains. We both went through our fair share of cough drops, especially when I ended up getting tonsillitis in New England. The Pepto Bismol came in handy after a particularly violent encounter with some dubious chicken wings in Oregon too.

When preparing your own Med Prep Kit, think about what you use regularly at home. You'll also want to consider the types of malaise you and your family find most bothersome and frequent. While a first aid kit is a good start, build the rest of your kit around your own reality. This chart provides some helpful examples:

| If You Experience... | Then Consider Packing... |
| --- | --- |
| Discomfort/Allergic Reactions to Bug Bites and Stings | - Instant ice packs<br>- Insect repellent<br>- Calamine lotion or hydrocortisone cream<br>- Antihistamines<br>- Oatmeal-based soap<br>- Epinephrine injectable for severe allergic reaction |
| Frequent sprains and strains | - Support braces for weak joints or painful areas<br>- Self-adhesive wraps<br>- Cream/lotion/ointment for sore muscles<br>- Battery operated TENS unit or other massage device, such as myofascial massage balls or foam roller<br>- Instant ice packs<br>- Extra towels or wash clothes for cold compresses<br>- Maximum strength pain reliever |
| Migraine Headaches | - Instant caffeine source<br>- Migraine relief medication (eg, Excedrin Migraine)<br>- Sleep mask to keep the light out<br>- Instant ice packs<br>- Ear plugs |
| Frequent Head Colds | - Daytime cold medication<br>- Nighttime cold medication<br>- Vitamin supplements<br>- Tea bags and honey (if you have a propane burner or other method for heating water quickly)<br>- Throat lozenges- heavy duty and regular strength |

As you read through this chart, you'll probably have moments of "Oh, I didn't think about that." and "That definitely doesn't apply to me." Those thoughts should be the basis for completing a chart like this that does resonate with the daily health needs of you and your family. Prepare for the unknown, but REALLY PREPARE for the known.

Amazingly, I didn't consider my frequent bouts of tonsillitis in the early months of Autumn until I was in complete agony somewhere in Vermont.

Instead of being prepared, I did exactly what I just told you not to do; I made Brad pull over at the first drug store we found, and I bought three different types of lozenges, two enormous bottles of NyQuil, a multipack of Puffs Plus infused with Vicks, dissolvable zinc tablets, a giant bottle of Vitamin C capsules, a box of Theraflu, and a little stuffed fish toy because I was feeling dumpy and it made me smile. I spent far more money than I needed to spend and bought a whole bunch of stuff I ended up using for a week at most. That meant we had to keep hauling it, which became redundant, and all it did after I started feeling better was take up space and get in the way.

Instead, I should have packed the one type of lozenge I use at home, quality tissues, zinc tablets, and NyQuil before we even left. The moment I started feeling a scratchy throat come on, I should've upped the Vitamin C. I don't regret the stuffed fish at all though. We named him Mr. Ferguson, and he's one of the van's mascots.

As far as storing your Med Prep Kit, I recommend giving it its own tote. That way, you'll know exactly where things are at all times, or at least where they should be. Make sure that this tote is always easily accessible too. As always, I recommend airtight and watertight totes to prevent infestation, mold, and dirt, since you want this kit to be in pristine condition at all times. Also, be sure to check the expiration dates on the creams and medications from time to time. They're not as effective if they're expired, and since time has no meaning on the road, you don't want to find this out in an emergency!

Before you even roll your van out on your first excursion, make sure you're prepared for the most common eventualities. While one of the main draws of van life is its unpredictable nature, there are certain health situations that you'll want to be able to head off quickly. Having a well-stocked, fully-intentional Med Prep Kit in your van is a great way to keep your everyday ouchies and yuckies at a minimum.

## What to Do When Things Get Worse

While most situations and symptoms can be treated on the go, you might occasionally find yourself completely wiped out by illness or injury.

Let me make this first part abundantly clear: That's okay. If you need to rest, please rest.

There seems to be this van life ego or bravada that stopping and resting somehow detracts from your experience. Perhaps it's because I'm older, or maybe it has to do with how many different breaks I had to take due to illness and injury, but there is absolutely no shame in taking time to let your body heal from whatever malady is currently haunting you. There's not a soul on this planet who wants you to share your germs if you happen to be ill, so just don't.

What to do when you're more than a little sick or hurt is directly related to your van setup. If you can successfully quarantine yourself within your van for a week or so while you wait for the worst to pass, that's ideal. Just make sure you have plenty of liquids, a nearby bathroom, adequate bedding, excellent air flow, and plenty of mindless activities to occupy yourself between nap times.

When you read the recommendations for any type of healing, "rest" always tops the list. Don't let some preconceived notion of what you ought to do take you away from what you need to do to help your body. Sure, you can push forward, but will you really enjoy it? As I mentioned earlier, I had a bout of tonsillitis in New England. I actually continued hiking through the symptoms until I nearly passed out on a trail. But, I insisted that we keep driving for several days. There were a few times I accompanied Brad in the van to the trailhead, and while he got to wander blissfully through the Adirondacks, traipse through Baxter State Park, and meander meaningfully through White Mountain National Forest, I laid in the back of the van intermittently sleeping and taking cold medicine.

So, why did I say, "Let's keep going!" even though I was miserable? Because I thought that's what van lifers do. Nowhere on social media was there a guidebook for what to do when your tonsils are the size of your fist. If I had been at home, I would've gone to my regular family doctor, gotten some medication, and snuggled into bed with hot tea and *The Price Is Right*. I felt like because I was on the road, I had to keep being on the road.

During my bout with tonsillitis, the local temperatures reached the mid-30s Fahrenheit at night. I was simultaneously too hot and too cold, depending on the time of day. We had no onboard electricity, running water, or toilet, which put serious limitations on my ability to have constant fluids. While I tried to make it work, we ended up finding a delightful - yet spartan - cottage in which I could spend a few nights recuperating. Being indoors and having the ability to fully rest, along with the amazing soup from a local cafe and a whole bunch of orange juice, did quite a bit to bring me back to health.

That is why, as I write this book, I strongly recommend rest to anyone who needs it. Unless you are on a dire timeline, don't feel that you need to push yourself to the breaking point to fulfill the "Ultimate Van Lifestyle."

Additionally, there is no shame in visiting a local Urgent Care. Just because you live in a van doesn't mean you're immortal! Urgent Care can be a great, low-cost stop for most general issues from a cough that won't go away to hiking accidents.

Before you go, make sure the Urgent Care you visit has the services you need. This may sound obvious, but I have personally experienced a city with multiple Urgent Care centers that all provide different services. To avoid the hassle of being transferred to the pricey emergency room (ER) or driving around looking for another location, be sure that if you're injured, the location you're heading to has digital x-ray services. If you're ill, make sure they can prescribe medications. If you can check the waitlist times online, all the better.

Sometimes, however, you actually need the ER. If you are experiencing any of the following symptoms, don't bother with looking up the ideal Urgent Care; instead, go immediately to the ER:

- Shortness of breath/difficulty breathing or swallowing
- Obvious bone breaks
- Bleeding that will not stop
- Head injury with loss of consciousness
- Unexplainable chest/abdominal pains
- Animal bites or attacks
- Stroke symptoms
- Fevers over 100 degrees Fahrenheit
- Burns to the hand or face, or greater than 3 inches in size
- When symptoms are persistent and don't respond to treatment

If you are living with a chronic condition, heed your care team's advice on when to head to the ER. If it's after hours for Urgent Care, yet symptoms are making it impossible to comfortably dwell in your van for the night, it is also reasonable to head to the Emergency Room for immediate care.

Perfect health is not a guarantee, and without the comforts of home, finding yourself under the weather for the first time while living on the road can be a bit of a shock to the system. However, it's not impossible to manage everything from chronic health conditions to the occasional cold or injury.

The two main things to factor in are preparedness and the ability to rest when you need to. During times of flare ups, illness, or injury, you might need to be more deliberate in your every move, but don't take this as a sign that the gods of the road want you to go home.

Over time, you'll have all of your self-care patterns down to a science. You'll learn new routines to replace those that you learned in your stationary home. You'll gain a better perspective of what you need to keep yourself well on the road. You'll probably make a few mistakes, but you'll definitely learn from them. From figuring out the best way to dispose of your used tissues and medical supplies, to storing your meds in places that make sense for how and when you take them, you'll need to pay a little more attention at first, but eventually your routine will emerge.

And when things take a turn for the worse? Don't be afraid to seek additional assistance. Allow yourself to stop and get the rest you need. You deserve to feel better quickly, so give your body the best chance it can to recuperate completely.

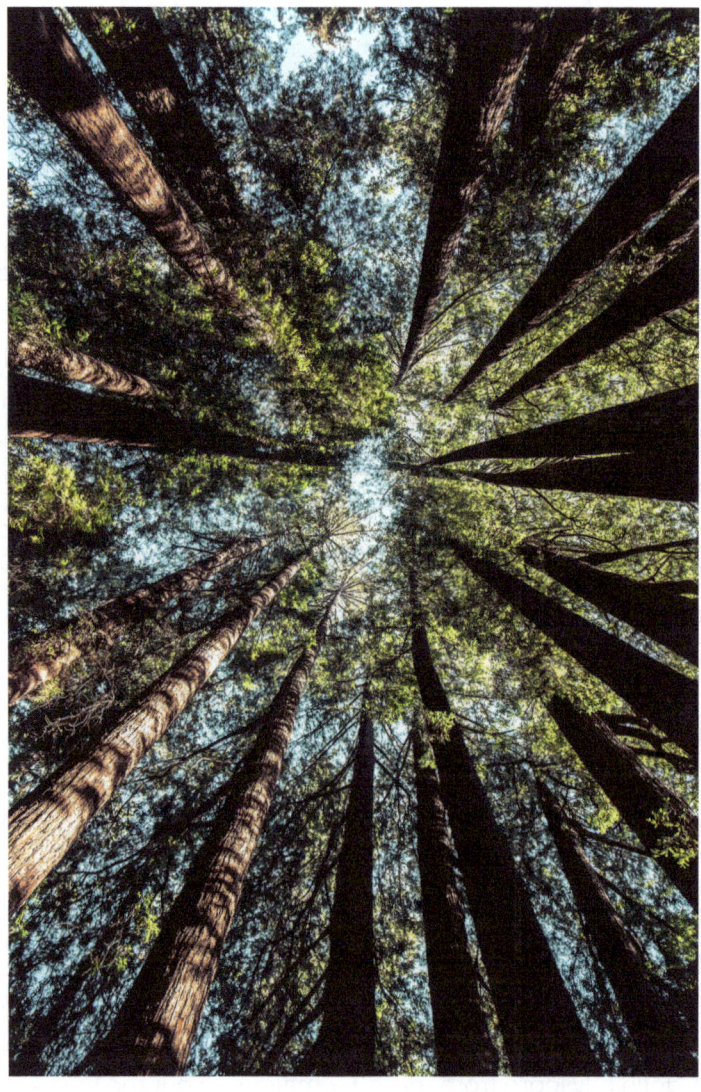

# Section 4: A Brief Section about Housekeeping and Hygiene

You might think housekeeping is a little out of place for a book that claims to address "health and wellness issues." This section will be shorter than the others because it would be impossible for me to tell you how to clean your personal living space with so many different cleaning methods, products, and needs based on your own system and the design of your van, skoolie, or RV.

Therefore, this is going to be a high-level overview about basic hygienic needs in a van. I have no doubt that each and every reader of this book is familiar with the need to clean all surfaces, change bed linens, do laundry, and bathe once in a while. These are skills that we're all proficient at to some degree or another.

When you take your life on the road, however, things change. There is no "pants chair." There is limited space for your intricate sorting method for clothing at various stages of the clean-to-dirty spectrum. If your floor is dirty, your feet will be dirty, and thus your bed will be dirty, and so on. There is limited room to avoid filth, so your ability to ignore a little momentary grossness is often compromised.

Imagine, if you will, a container of leftover soup. Perhaps you take this leftover soup out of the cooler in an attempt to reach a water bottle below it. Maybe you forget that the soup is sitting next to the cooler and go to bed. The consequence for this minor mishap, as Brad and I can attest, is your van smelling like soup for 3-4 days. This is compounded by a devout following of insects, despite driving with all possible windows open and creating a wind vortex in the back.

Cleanliness matters in a van. Whether you just want to be able to sleep without wondering what that stink is, or you're intent on managing allergies and preventing growth of any nasty bacteria around the van, keep in mind that just a little bit of cleaning can go a long way. Let's take a quick look at some of the simple things you can do to keep a tidy home on the road.

## Chapter 1: Basic Van Cleanliness

We should all acknowledge that a van is not going to be an antiseptic vacuum. If you have the windows or doors open even for a millisecond, the wind can blow in dust, pollen, leaves, or tiny insects. Unless you are camping on the production floor for a major cleaning product company, there will be a dusting of the outdoors in your van at all times. If you can write your name in the sand on the dashboard, it might be time to make a few adjustments!

First, consider bugs. Most of the insects and arachnids you meet along the way have an important job to do within their natural ecosystem. They also love getting a free ride with an all-you-can-eat buffet. More relevant to the matter at hand, they can bring with them some really unpleasant diseases, such as Lyme disease from ticks, or West Nile Virus and Zika from mosquitoes.

Make sure your screens and filters are all in good shape at all times, and that any free-standing screens fit tightly against your windows. If you use mosquito netting around your bed or sleeping areas, make sure there aren't any gaping holes, and repair or replace them as needed.

Check your entire food supply regularly for any invaders. In my experience, there is no such thing as "just one fly." So, make sure you're looking in the bins, the cupboards, the cooler, and the refrigerator daily to ensure no one is getting a free meal or reproducing in your important nutrients.

If you do find signs of unwanted arthropodic company, my first recommendation is to isolate the affected item or items. If you can wrap it in a grocery bag and drop it off in a trash can at a gas station or rest stop, all the better. If the infestation is in a larger object, such as a mattress or pillow, the first thing to do is isolate the source. Get the object out of the van, and wrap it in plastic- for example, those huge mattress moving bags can be really helpful in situations like this. I won't go so far as to recommend you carry one with you at all times, but keep this in mind as a "just in case" scenario.

Treatment of an infestation depends entirely on the type of insect involved and how far you're personally willing to go to get involved with this battle. Sometimes you can treat the object with commercially available chemicals and move on; other bugs require a greater level of finesse. I will say that if you decide to take matters into your own hands, remember first the impact of what you're doing to the area around you, the native wildlife, and your own family or travel companions. Letting off a flea bomb in the skoolie might make sense on paper, but where are the fumes going to go? Where are you going to do this so that it doesn't have a negative impact on land, air, water, or other wildlife? Don't say "the parking lot of the Wal-Mart where I buy the bomb," because that is the sort of thing that will go viral on social media in milliseconds. Insect infestations are very inconvenient and definitely have a very high "yuck" factor, but you can't have knee-jerk reactions when you live in a van. Be deliberate and plan carefully.

One way to mitigate potential insect problems is to keep all of your van surfaces as clean as possible. That means wiping down any counters or shelves, sweeping the floor, shaking out the bedding and rugs to rid them of any crumbs, and keeping up with all of your dishes.

Possibly the easiest way to incorporate this type of complete cleaning overhaul into your day is to make it part of the evening meal routine. After finishing supper, immediately wash and dry your dishes and store them back in their tote, cupboard, or drawer. If you have a sink, wash it out. Wipe down all of the counters or table tops, and use a hand broom to get the crumbs off of any indoor seating. Some people feel fine with doing a thorough sweep of the floor before closing up, but I personally prefer to do a quick mopping. Since the floor space in my van measures about 4 feet by three feet, this does not require exceptional effort- I can use a designated floor sponge and the leftover dish water. So long as there's nothing really gross or stinky floating in there, I can simply lean into the van through the door to quickly wipe down the floor.

Bedding can be tricky, depending on your rig's setup. If you're able to, remove linens from your bed each day and give them a good air fluff. That should give you enough of a chance to disturb anything attempting to nest in it and allow you to inspect it for holes and swarms. I know this sounds terrible, but in your attempt to integrate with nature, nature will often make the first move.

Though it may be very tempting, do not spray bug spray inside the cabin, and especially not on your bedding. Most bug sprays stick to the skin via an oil base, so not only will they leave greasy streaks on your surfaces, but dirt and dust will also adhere to these sticky spots, giving you an equally bad time. There are some natural ways to dissuade insects from joining you on the road, such as vinegar, garlic, and citronella-based products. Just make sure you can live with the smell, and that storing your solution isn't more of a pain than a few irritating insects!

**Chapter 2: Laundry Day!**
When I asked my van buddies the number one thing they forget about when it came to chores and tidiness, almost all of them answered with "laundry day." At home, it's generally pretty easy to toss your dirty socks and tees in a hamper or dark corner and forget about them for a week or so. In a van, you probably have two days maximum before the socks in the corner start to haunt you, depending on the weather.

Hand-in-hand with keeping the van clean is coming up with an appropriate way to manage your laundry. This can be extra important when you're outdoors for long periods of time, as the pollen and dirt you encounter out there can easily trek into the van with you. Plus, sweat is one of those stenches that gets more pungent with time.

How you choose to do your laundry is entirely up to you. Some people like the convenience of stopping at a laundromat every so often. There are plenty of upsides to this plan. Many laundromats sell single-use detergent packets, which means you don't have to haul a bulky potential leak hazard around with you. Many laundromats also have amenities that we miss on the road such as running water, cold drink machines, air conditioning, and free WiFi. If your van is missing any of these, it might be a fine idea to spend a few hours basking in civilization in a laundromat.

Others prefer to go boondocking and stay boondocking. You can absolutely do your laundry from your van, as long as you have enough water for washing and rinsing. Roof racks are a fantastic place to let your clean clothes naturally air dry too; just make sure you firmly weigh your clothing down. Otherwise, you'll find yourself chasing your unmentionables through the wilderness as they dry and catch the wind.

If you choose to do your laundry from the van, I strongly urge you to be cautious about the type of detergent you use. The suds you dump onto the ground will be shared with all the flora and fauna in the area, so it's important to choose products that are non-toxic and environmentally friendly. The same goes for all of your cleaning products, shampoos, and soaps. Look for words like "biodegradable" on the labels, or check out a few tutorials online for making your own nature-friendly cleaning products. Don't worry, there are a few helpful links on this topic in the Resources section!

**Chapter 3: Clean Van, Clean You**
Now that I've gently eased you into the topic of basic van cleanliness, let's touch for a moment on personal hygiene.

On one hand, what does it matter what you smell like, or what kind of funk dwells deep within your armpits? You're alone or with your closest mates in the middle of nowhere, so is it important?

Well, yes and no. If you choose to take dirt baths and let your hair go completely *au naturel*, that is completely your prerogative. No judgment here. However, I will ask you to consider sponging up before and after you hit civilization.

You see, dirt itself is actually pretty harmless, compared to all the gross stuff humans spread around with their hands, their feet, and even with involuntary acts like breathing, yawning, sneezing, and coughing. When you touch something, all of the microscopic stuff living on that particular surface uses your body as a free ride. If you have an open wound, then touch your face, those microscopic particles use the opportunity to take a tour of your body.

Most of the stuff we touch is no big deal. Even if it isn't, our bodies are designed to fight off infections. Your immune system is equipped with natural warriors in the form of white blood cells, antibodies, mucus, and more to attack the invading virus, bacteria, fungus, or other toxins. Antibodies are produced as a reaction to acquired defense, so the first time your body encounters a particular germ, it may react poorly.

Want an easy way to prevent infection? Wash your hands. That may sound really familiar, but it bears repeating. Washing your body also gives you the opportunity to rid your skin of the bacteria, oils, and dead skin cells that are constantly piling up. Normally, that's no big deal, because your body is designed to take care of itself. But if you fall on a trail and scrape your knee, that bacteria is right there, ready to jump in and make a ruckus of your immune system. Don't let it. At the very minimum, keep wounds and compromised areas clean while your body does its job healing.

Furthermore, be mindful of what you track back into the van. When your skin and hair have more oil build up than usual, it's easy for germs and dirt to cling to your body and hitch a ride in your van. Again, that's rarely a big deal - except for when you're mingling with other people or environments.

Take, for example, White-Nose Syndrome, caused by a fungus that enjoys cold, damp, dark areas. White-Nose Syndrome affects hibernating bats. You may be wondering what that has to do with your human, van-life bathing habits. It's all about travel! White-Nose Syndrome has killed millions of bats since it was first identified in 2006, and it is theorized that it is spread minimally by bats travelling from cave system to cave system. Instead, it's largely spread by humans walking through cave systems, getting spores and guano on their shoes, and then walking in those shoes through another bat population, spreading the dangerous spores.

To mitigate the issue and keep the delicate ecosystem of caves in balance, many cave systems have installed disinfecting mats at the entrances and/or exits of their tour areas.

Similar logic applies to you, your natural biology, and the places you visit. The hiker's creed is "take nothing but photos; leave nothing but footprints," keep that in mind with your own personal hygiene and your interaction with local populations.

In the same line of thought, brushing your teeth in a van can be challenging without running water. It's a highly recommended activity for maintaining the health of your teeth and gums, and preventing infection originating in the mouth. You'll likely want to take care of your teeth when you're far from a dentist.

One suggestion is to keep a separate water bottle for clean water and rinse water. Rinse water can be captured in a tub and disposed of at any public restroom with a regular septic system. It's a bit more low-tech than a grey water system, but easy enough since brushing your teeth generally doesn't require a lot of water. You may wish to replace your toothbrush more frequently, or as many intrepid boondockers do, boil it from time to time, since the amount of rinsing you'll be able to do without running water is somewhat limited. I can't speak for the actual efficacy of boiling your toothbrush in the woods, so I'll leave that decision entirely up to you!

What about floss, and mouthwash? Absolutely wonderful considerations when it comes to maintaining dental hygiene, but not exactly environmentally friendly. Floss, for example, should absolutely not be discarded anywhere in the wild, as it can be harmful to wildlife. Instead, I recommend wrapping used floss in a bit of napkin and adding it to your regular trash. As long as you dispose of your trash frequently, it shouldn't create a noticeable stench.

Mouthwash is tricky, because you definitely don't want to accidentally re-use that. If you have a way to deposit your used swishes in the black water, that's ideal. If you choose to only use potent mouthwash when you're in a public bathroom, that's another great option. If you need to use a regular mouthwash - either medicated or at a doctor's recommendation - the most important thing is that you don't accidentally introduce it to ground water or make it available to wildlife. This may mean carting around a well-labeled spitoon of sorts for the time being. Just be sure to dump, rinse, and sanitize it regularly to avoid creating a small, portable biohazard of your own!

I'm going to great pains here to avoid inadvertently shaming anyone's personal hygiene routine; however, I did want to include the topic to provide tips to those who haven't considered the potential challenges. Many new van lifers don't think about the possible complications of trying to brush your teeth without running water, in the dark, while coyotes howl somewhere much closer than you would prefer. I bring these topics up simply to give those who are new to van life- or at least boondocking - some helpful ideas. Also, I want to remind those who have lost that sense of naivete through experience that cleanliness is still an important aspect of overall wellness!

## Section 5: Mental Health Matters

Most of us turn to van life because there is something about stationary dwelling that just isn't "doing it" for us. Sometimes, there are unignorable mental health aspects at play that help drive our decision.

Perhaps the whole home/work routine isn't working. Maybe you feel life is passing you by too quickly. There might be high levels of anxiety caused by doing the same thing, every day. Maybe the reason you chose van life is because you needed to be outside with every bit of your soul, and let's be honest – you've sacrificed a lot to make your soul happy.

So, when you wake up in your beautiful van, to a 360-degree vista of exotic beauty, doing exactly what you want to be doing, how can you possibly feel depressed or anxious? If you're reading this book from the comfort of a house, apartment, condo, or other permanent dwelling, this idea may not make sense. For those who have been on the road for a bit, you've probably already experienced symptoms of road fatigue, anxiety, and depression, all related to the huge change you've just made in your life.

I have good news: you're absolutely not the first and only person who has ever felt this way. On the other hand, I have not-so-great news: these feelings don't just "go away."

In this section, I'll take a look at some common mental health issues that may pop up on the road. Even if you have never suffered from mental illness in the past, you are still human. Humans have emotions, and our minds and bodies respond to stress in ways that will never cease to shock and amaze us – even good stress! I fully hope everyone reading this book has a safe, enjoyable adventure, but if you do feel like something is not quite right on a mental or emotional level, this section is for you.

Please know that mental health is just as important as physical health and can even impact your immune response, sleep patterns, energy levels, and more. Do not ignore any changes in your thought patterns or emotions.

As mentioned before, this book is not intended to take the place of your regular therapist or counselor, and the advice of your professional team should always take priority!

NOTE:

- If you are currently in a decent place with your mental health and ready to read more about potential mental health challenges when you're on the road, go ahead and read on.

- If you may be triggered by reading about mental health right now, go ahead and jump to Section 6. I promise I'm not offended. Come back to this section when you're in a better space, and look after your own safety right now.
-
- If you are in crisis and may be a danger to yourself or others, or have a plan to cause harm, please put the book down and reach out for help. There is no shame in asking for help when you need it. If you can't get in touch with an understanding friend or family member right now, visit [https://suicidepreventionlifeline.org/](https://suicidepreventionlifeline.org/), or call the Lifeline at 1-800-273-8255.

When you're ready, read on to learn more about some of the unique challenges van living can have on our brains and how to keep your chin up and your outlook positive while dealing with them.

### Chapter 1: The Reality of Road Fatigue

There are different types of discomfort that fall under the umbrella term of "road fatigue." Sometimes it's that zombie-like feeling you have when you've completed a long day of endless driving. You might be physically stiff, extremely sleepy, and devoid of thought or feeling. You even see headlights when you close your eyes!

Generally speaking, this level of fatigue will wear off quickly once you've had some rest, mental stimulation, or a nutritious meal. The symptoms you experience are simply the brain's way of saying that it's overloaded with the same stimuli, and it's time to switch things up a bit.

**But What If It's Worse Than That?**

The next level involves feeling stiff and sleepy, but you might be extra grumpy, too. Nothing sounds "good," and you're kind of mad about it. You can hear yourself whining like an overtired child, and you're actively embarrassed for anyone who's putting up with you right now. Still, you can't stop feeling irritated, even after a long rest or a break. Even when nothing particularly stressful is happening in the moment, you might find yourself thinking about something that made you feel cranky not too long ago, just to have a good reason for feeling the way you do.

If you're feeling this way right now, try this exercise:

1. Close your eyes (not while driving!)
2. Take several deep, cleansing breaths until you no longer feel actively cranky. Feeling tense is fine – that's an improvement.
3. Can you think of a time when you felt like this, even just a little bit? Maybe it was in school, when you had a whole bunch of things due all at once, and your friends were being weird, and your family was on your case about making a life for yourself. Perhaps it was at work, when it felt like literally everyone was in your face about something you had to do NOW, NOW, NOW! It could have been in conjunction with getting prepared for a big holiday gathering or a huge vacation.
4. Don't replay that memory too much. Instead, fast forward to the part where you felt better. Chances are good that there was some event or date that occurred, after which all the pressure let up and you could go back to your normal levels of stress. Once the pressure released, so did all the negative feelings, right?

Now, open your eyes. In the next three minutes, you're going to get really grumpy again, because you'll realize you don't have any magic date or event that will cause you to feel less stressed out, and how can you possibly relax when you don't even know where you're going to find your next meal?

This may not make sense right now, but this is actually really good news. You're admitting that you're stressed out. Transitioning to van life is stressful. Even if you are fully physically prepared, your brain may not have gotten the memo.

There is a specific type of stress that occurs when you abruptly change routine on yourself. Think about how hard it is to start waking up an hour earlier every day. Then look around you. You have taken everything you've known, for your entire life, and put it in the rearview mirror. There are no bubble baths. There is no pizza delivery. You have probably gotten pretty good at going to the bathroom outside in the dark. This is not your normal!

This level of stress has been building and building. And just like everything else in this world, your emotional threshold for pressure can only bend so much before something has to give.

I actually had this epiphany while watching Old Faithful erupt at Yellowstone National Park. If you haven't been, I highly recommend it. Geysers erupt due to the relentless building pressure of steam released from water boiling far underground. When the pressure becomes too high, fountains of boiling water burst through the ground with incredible force. As the water cools below the boiling point, the eruption stops, and everything goes back to a calm, quiet state.

You are very much like a geyser, only less boiling water, and more complicated emotions. Your mind can handle stress. It accepts it as a reality. Logically, you know what's coming and probably have a good idea of how you'll react. When things go slightly sideways as you start your van adventure, you brush them off. It's no big deal. This is what you wanted. When you find yourself staring at the ceiling of the van at midnight, wishing you could talk to your best friend, you tell yourself you're doing something so much better. Squelch the feeling, and go to sleep. You chose to leave them behind, after all. This is not a healthy model to follow, and builds the pressure under your emotional geyser.

Stress can take a really heavy toll on your mental and emotional health. Stop trying to talk yourself out of your emotions. You're allowed to miss your friends. It makes perfect sense that you want to go home. Our brains and bodies thrive on routine, even if we don't agree with the concept. Yes, you wanted to do this. Yes, it was the best idea for you. But don't fool yourself that you should be proud and happy "instead of" mopey. It is not "failure" if you aren't feeling as much van life gusto on the third month as you did on the third day.

If you find yourself feeling grumpy, cranky, crunchy, indecisive, anti-social, or extra moody in any way, assess your honest stress level. What you need to do is simultaneously let yourself have feelings and find ways to direct that negative energy into something that will benefit you. Start with the exercise I've outlined. Maybe you don't have a date or event that will release this pressure, but you can create one.

Cry because you miss your friends. Then schedule a video call with as many of them as possible. Look at your itinerary and find the best time to go visit them. You have wheels – use them!

Miss lying in bed and watching television? Find a decent, inexpensive hotel for the night. Brad and I were able to score a fabulous hotel room in New Mexico for less than what camping spots in the area cost. Was it a penthouse suite? No, but it was clean, the sheets were cool, the air conditioning and the shower worked, and I actually cried because I saw a commercial on television for the first time in three months.

Your mind gives you plenty of red flags when the pressure starts to build, and since there is no shame in listening to what your body needs, pay attention to these signals. The final step in the exercise outlined earlier is to close your eyes again, and ask yourself honestly, what do you need? A break? A hug? A meal that reminds you of home? Once you've identified what you need to help you cope with the pressure you're feeling, set a course to make it happen. Chances are likely that you'll soon discover that things like spilling water on your seats will stop sending you into a tantrum.

### The Side Effects of Having Too Much Time to Think

There's also a type of road fatigue that I call "The Backdoor Panics." That is in no way a medical term, but the best way I can describe the sensation.

At some point in your life, you've probably experienced this scenario. You're fast asleep. Suddenly, you wake up. Your pets might have made noise, you had to go to the bathroom, or you discovered your sleeping position was giving you a cramp. Either way, it was completely involuntary. You make all the necessary adjustments again, and before your head can hit the pillow, the Backdoor Panic appears. Out of nowhere, you remember the second grade science fair. Specifically, you remember how you forgot the science fair, because you thought it was still a week away. Chaos ensued, and you ended up with some half-cooked "project" accompanied by stammering and stuttering your way through a moment of epic failure. Suddenly, you've gone from a pleasant, restful state, to heart-racing, cold-sweating, full-blown anxiety!

Maybe it wasn't your second grade science fair, though this is a true story from my own past. I share this as an example of a real Back Door Panic I had somewhere on the road in Texas. I happened to see a mouse skeleton, which reminded me of the skeletons I used to collect as a kid, which started in second grade, and, well, you can see where this is headed. Regardless, this is not the sort of thing that should be keeping anyone awake at night. It's over. It's done. If it was the cataclysmic event that set off the rest of our collective destiny, there's still nothing that can be done about it, especially not in the middle of the night.

But this is exactly how the Back Door Panic works. It shows up when your mind is relaxed, and you have nothing but empty hours to dwell on all sorts of terrible things.

What does this have to do with van living? When you live in a van, you will have plenty of quiet, empty time to fill with thoughts. When you're feeling particularly stressed or vulnerable, your brain will tenderly associate all of the times you felt lousy, and run it past you in a never-ending loop of failure. Basically, your bad feelings come in through the "backdoor" of your mind, and as a result, you may start to feel super depressed or unbelievably anxious.

The fact that a complete stranger is explaining this phenomenon to you should give you hope that you are not alone. Even if you're feeling pretty great about everything, those long stretches on the road can be very tricky for the mind. I strongly recommend preparing adequate distractions, such as music, podcasts, audio books - anything to keep you less focused on the dark recesses of your memory.

If you're not in the driver's seat, you have even more options available. As long as you have a way to keep your phone charged, indulge in some phone games. If you're feeling lonely, hit up some forums or social media groups in a niche you love. As a word of caution, though, don't forget that social media groups can sometimes be incredibly volatile. If you're feeling particularly vulnerable, back away from any outlet, group, or post that is making you feel stressed and explosive. Don't let someone else's mindless words trigger your emotional state. If it's too late and the damage is done, my best recommendation is to reach out to someone sympathetic, such as a friend who also shares your interests.

For those who are travelling in pairs or as a family, I encourage you to be open with your traveling companions about how you're feeling. Even a skoolie is a very small, contained area, and your change in attitude and mood will be noticed. By communicating your feelings, you'll prevent a chain reaction of discontent, unease, and even paranoia. Plus, there's something about sharing your negative emotions that seems to defuse them a bit.

Success is not measured by how many consecutive nights you stay in your van. Your self-worth is not determined by how many meals you've eaten by yourself in the woods. Snuggling down in a hotel room with a delivery pizza isn't a sign of weakness or failure. Instead, these are signs that your mind needs a break, and that you are honoring that need. While it would be great if we could all just handle infinite amounts of stress without cracking, that is not reality. Honor your signs of stress and anxiety, and take care of them before you become a full geyser.

## Chapter 2: Finding and Continuing Mental Health Care on the Road

For some reason, therapy and counseling have gotten a bad reputation as an act of desperation or failure. Honestly, I don't understand this concept. If you've ever been to a Happy Hour event with your coworkers and complained about your boss, if you've talked to your spouse about a friend who is getting on your nerves, or if you've sat with a best friend over a cup of coffee and spilled all of your secrets... you have essentially completed the steps required for a therapy session.

The point of therapy and counseling is to talk through your issues with someone who is qualified to help guide your train of thoughts to help you focus on potential solutions, changes, or coping mechanisms. That's it. A therapist will not "cure you," but they will ease the burden of stress and pressure. A weekly or monthly session is usually the perfect opportunity to vent all of your frustrations while an empathetic therapist or counselor helps you dive into why you're frustrated, what caused you to react negatively, and come up with some ways to deal with your emotions.

When you're on the road, however, you can't just pop into your therapist's office once a week. If you've been in therapy for awhile, you'll know that freshly gutted feeling that comes with knowing you'll have to take your mental health into your own hands. Thankfully, technology has made it so that we can continue getting the help we need, even when we're on the road.

If one-on-one sessions are your jam, then consider online therapy options. You can choose from video conferencing, texting, emailing, and even phone calls with your designated therapist. Some programs allow for anytime-contact and assistance, while others offer flexible scheduling. This means that as long as you have a smartphone or other workable device and a clear signal, you can connect with a trained professional who can help you talk it out.

If you absolutely love the care professionals you have now, it can't hurt to approach them about telehealth. Before the COVID-19 outbreak of 2020, this was an almost unheard-of practice. However, with in-person visits limited due to potential spread of disease, more and more established practices are open to contacting patients through video calls.

You may prefer more interactive group sessions instead. It can be very helpful to talk through your concerns in a room full of sympathetic, like-minded individuals who have had similar experiences. You may think that hitting the road means leaving group sessions behind, but you'll be surprised to find that many cities, towns, and even villages have meetings that anyone is welcome to attend.

Granted, if you have anxiety about new social settings, you might not feel very cavalier about walking into a room full of complete strangers and airing all of your deepest secrets. If that sounds like the last possible thing you might ever want to do, take heart- online virtual group sessions exist for exactly this reason.

You might be a little concerned about the privacy aspect, especially if you're sitting in a van with the windows down, trying to be heard over a dubious phone connection. For that reason, I recommend doing a little scouting before you join in. Some of the best online support groups will have not just meetings, but also a forum or group page on social media where you can chat with others in the group and get to know each other. The pressure is minimal. If you don't like it, then unsubscribe, unfollow, block, delete, or whatever combination of words that particular forum uses to leave that group. There are thousands of communities out there if you're willing to do the legwork to find a group that most fits your needs.

Having a support system on the road is crucial for anyone who might be feeling extra stress, anxiety, or depression related to the massive life changes related to leaving "home" behind in favor of van life. While not every person who cares about you will understand why you're on the road, nearly everyone will appreciate how much change can impact our emotional and mental health. You need someone in your corner who is willing to listen, guide, and instigate coping or change - whichever is needed to help you find a healthier outlook to your stressors.

## Chapter 3: When It Becomes Too Much

There may be a time when you start to feel a certain way. If you were still living in a house with a 9-5 job, you'd say you were feeling burnt out, and that you needed a vacation. But here you are, living in a van, essentially living an eternal vacation. How can you possibly be burnt out?

As I've mentioned repeatedly, van life is stressful. On top of that, regular stress doesn't end just because you don't have a mailbox and a driveway. You may not have to deal with your daily commute, but traffic is still a reality. You don't have to appear in an office, but income is still helpful. You won't have to come face-to-face with that annoying relative, but chances are good that they still remember your phone number. Stress is everywhere, and for all of us, sometimes too much is just *way too much*.

When this happens, take a reverse vacation. Go hunker down with some friends or family members you love. You'll be surprised at how cool people feel with your van parked in their driveway. (On a related note - if you have a skoolie, you might need to make parking arrangements before you try parking in a suburban housing development!) A few days of indoor plumbing, climate control, cable television, and a microwave might be what your soul is craving in order to feel like balance is restored.

Alternately, you can tap out and plant for a bit. This means going deep into a boondocking area, where there's no phone signal, no WiFi, no people. It's just you, nature, and your van. The first time you do this, you may want to prepare beforehand by stopping at a grocery store, making sure you've got plenty of ice and clean clothes, and ensuring your spare tire and Med Prep and repair kits are all good to go.

Once you've got all the necessities, find the most intimidating camping spot you can find and hang out there for a few days. Meditate. Journal. Read. Draw. Create. Hike. Whatever brings you solace and serenity and keeps your mind from spiraling in on itself – this is the time to do it.

On the entirely opposite side of the coin, maybe you need the rush of city life. If you've been living in a metropolitan area your entire life, and you've just spent two months boondocking, the solitude might be causing you stress. If the funds are available, put the van in long-term parking, and have a city adventure.

I will fully admit that I have done this. After spending weeks in the deserts of the American West, Brad and I decided we needed a change of pace, so we booked a trip to Hawaii. We stayed in a hotel, rotted on the beach, ordered room service, and did a whole bunch of super-touristy things that we would usually laugh at. But it worked. When we came back to the van, we weren't upset at all about the sand in our pants. We didn't mind that weird soup smell that would never go away. We felt more prepared for deeper boondocking because we saw the city lights and felt that much more comfortable with the stars for having done so.

Van life is not a black-and-white sort of adventure. You can come and go. You can stop and rest, or keep moving. The whole point of van life is to custom tailor your daily experience to feed your soul, which includes your mind and your emotions. There's no such thing as "cheating" or "failing." Do whatever you need to do to keep yourself healthy and fulfilled to live your very best van life.

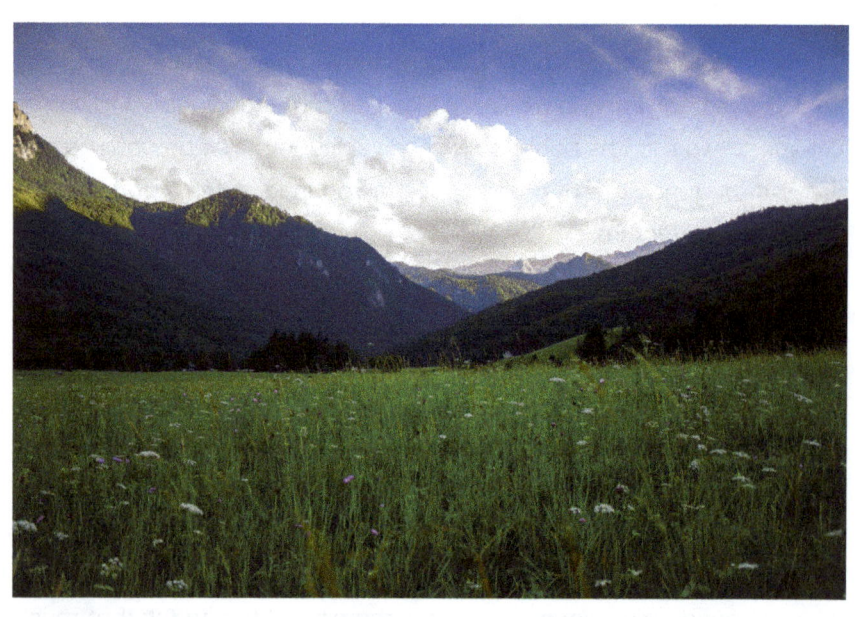

# Health and Wellness in 2020: Special Notes About COVID-19 Considerations

I started planning this book long before the COVID-19 pandemic was on the world's collective radar. When I first started making notes, I included all of the bits about being careful to not pick up and spread strange diseases due to being a traveler. I had no idea what was in store with a global pandemic on the horizon.

When I hit the road in 2018, I was startled by how often I got the sniffles or a little sore throat. Was it allergies? Was it related to incredibly different climates to my muggy and volatile Ohio weather? Or was I coming down with a swift bug? Without a full medical laboratory and an advanced degree in medicine, I had no way of knowing. So, I did what I could to boost my immune system with good nutrition, exercise, and sleep. I also kept the van clean, and practiced a reasonable amount of hand-washing. We had disinfectant wipes in the van for any questionable moments and hand sanitizer at the ready. At the same time, Brad and I thought nothing of taking our toothbrush into a rest station or fast food restaurant to clean up quickly with some running water. There were no masks and we regularly visited heavily congested parks and museums.

The current COVID-19 landscape is much different. Reservations are required to get into National Parks and museums - if they're even open at all. Camping in organized sites is extremely limited, and those that do have bathrooms may no longer allow access to them. In some states, restaurants are open for take-out only and you must patiently wait in line for the chance to enter a grocery store.

In some ways, van life is less stressful. Everything we need is artfully contained within a single space. Hardly anyone touches our surfaces except us, and self-quarantine is pretty much our way of life.

In other ways, living in a van can be much more stressful. Entertainment options run out quickly. Spontaneous travel to new locations is limited, as reservations to enter parks and campsites often sell out months in advance.

Travelling between states is, in several cases, prohibited. Attractions you've been eager to visit may be closed, and nearly every public event has been cancelled or very strictly limited.

Thankfully, one thing that has not been cancelled is nature. The trees are still growing, the winds are still blowing, and the flowers are still blooming. As I'm writing this section, the West Coast is currently on fire, and the East Coast is getting pummeled by hurricanes. So, that phrase might be slightly tinged with shades of hope, but until the actual end of the planet, nature is not officially done.

Before you set out each day, I do recommend taking a look at travel advisories to see where you're permitted to go based on your most recent location. I understand that no one wants to purposefully spread disease. I further understand that van lifers are, by nature, a rebellious sort. Different states have different requirements and penalties for not obeying their travel requirements. If you have the choice to go anywhere you want, choose a place where the risk is less. Quite frankly, every van lifer should be exquisitely prepared to quarantine in their van for fourteen days!

There's a little phrase that sticks in my mind at times like this: Calculated Risk. There are a lot of contagious diseases out there, and that's why we should all be exercising a significant amount of caution. This is especially so if we have a lifestyle in which we meet and share space with a lot of different people in rapid succession. Van dwellers should already be washing their hands thoroughly and using hand sanitizer frequently.

When Brad and I first hit the road in 2018, we each had a pocket-sized hand sanitizer on our person at all times, plus a container of sanitizing wipes in the back. Neither of us are anywhere near the stereotype of "germaphobes," either. I grew up riding horses and his family had a sheep farm. We're simply aware that gross stuff can get on your hands, and rather than getting it in your mouth or where you sleep, it's best to clean it off.

Masks are difficult. I get it. I'm constantly running into things because I can't see over the edges, sweating under them, and fidgeting under them. They're not something I love, but something I deal with because they let me do what I love, like visit breweries and try new foods. Again, always with calculated risk. Brad and I tend to visit places at non-peak times, request to sit in very low-traffic areas, and get take-out whenever possible. Sharing a growler of ale and a woodfired pizza in the back of the van while camped for the night is an absolute ideal type of evening for me, and totally worth wearing a mask to make it all happen.

Really, many van folks are already social distancing champions. We live a sort of lifestyle in which not being able to see what nearby campers are up to is actually a treat. I remember finding this prime boondocking location in Arizona - it was just us, a single tree, and the sunset. And then an RV rolled up. "Oh, come ON!" Brad lamented into the sunset. "How did you even find us?" That's the sort of attitude I've found prevalent amongst many van lifers. We've got a hearty sense of community, but if we wanted to hang out with people all the time, we would've stayed in the suburbs.

Therefore, in the name of calculated risk, I encourage you to hang on to your van lifer ideals. Yes, life was much more interesting when we could stop and talk to everyone we encountered on the trails. You still can ask the locals the best places to check out. From a distance of 6 feet, of course, and while wearing a mask. You might think these are paranoia-fueled rules, but basic outdoorsmanship and survival skills are rooted in taking precautions that mutually benefit you and nature. If you can run your backpack up a tree to discourage night predators from stopping by for a snack, you can also slip a mask on before interacting with people face-to-face.

And then, when you've reached the apex of an incredible hike, or found that boondocking spot where no one can find you, you can slip off your mask, take several deep breaths, and absolutely revel in the delicious moments of being a nature-loving, solitude-seeking van lifer.

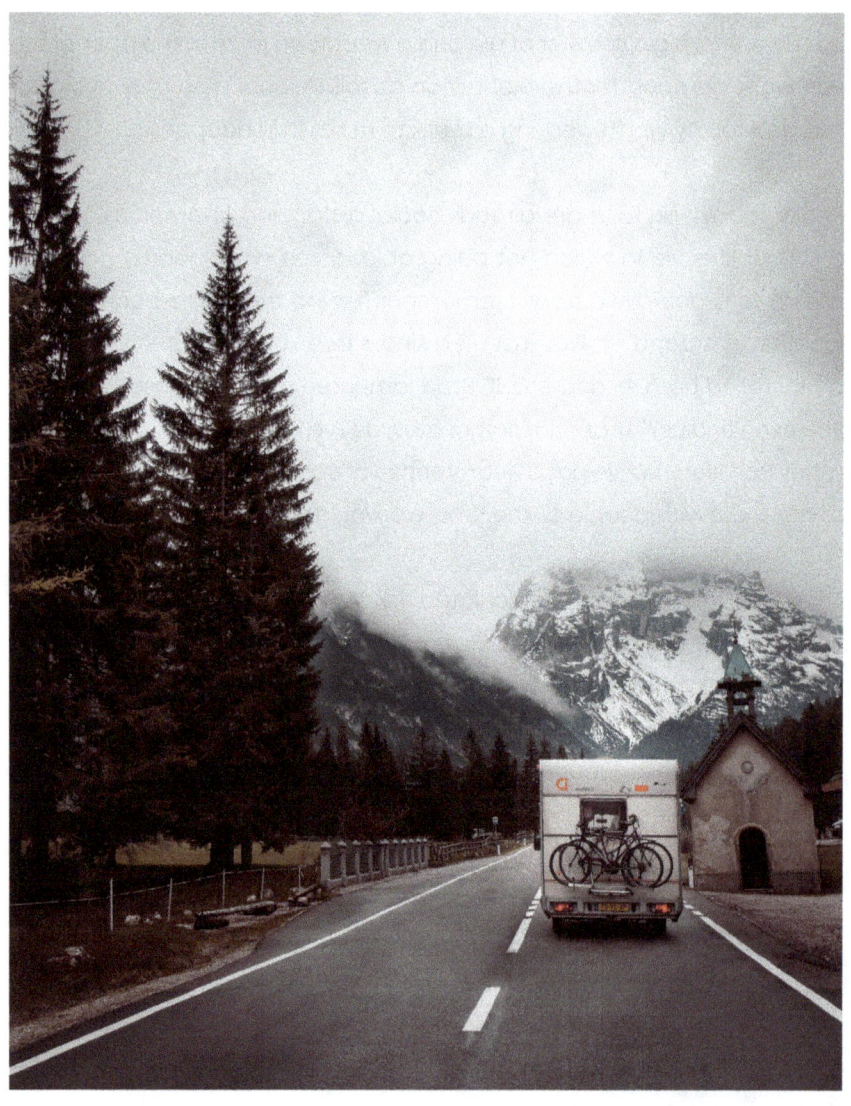

# Conclusion

At the very beginning of this book, I promised you that there wouldn't be any overwhelming revelations, and I hope that remains true. My goal in writing this book was to remove some of the surprises and stigma, and provide a whole heap of reminders and tips for staying healthy while you're on the road.

For our inaugural van trip, Brad and I started out in late April. We had a great run until September, when it seemed like we were getting hit with back-to-back colds. At first, we were terribly stubborn and tried to push through, but that was a very, very bad idea in retrospect. If we had paused until we were feeling better, we could have easily extended our trip and really enjoyed the opportunities that were just beyond the doors of the van. Instead, we ended up crawling back to home base in mid-October, worn out, and carrying an impressive-but-unnecessary array of cold medicines and throat lozenges.

Is this a cautionary tale? Not entirely. I can't stop you from picking up minor illnesses, and I'm literally the last person who can prevent you from getting injured. I don't want you to give up your dreams, and I definitely think you should go base-jumping if that's your life's dream. I want you to exercise caution, but I want you to have fun in your feral new lifestyle, after all!

What I'm hoping this book does is open your eyes to a little bit of the reality that is van life. The models on social media make it look so clean and airy, beautiful and decadent. The "beautiful" part is accurate. "Airy" can be, too, if the weather is nice. But clean? Decadent? Those parts are entirely up to you, and in my opinion, are also mutually exclusive.

I encourage each person reading this book to take care of yourself, whether that means following the recommendations and tips presented in this book to the letter, or just paying attention to the cues your body is feeding you. I want you to know that if you are feeling a certain type of bad - whether that's in your body, in your mind, or in your emotions - there are things you can do to help yourself feel a little better.

If you haven't experienced life on the road yet, you might find many of these tips to be common sense and basic knowledge. Before you roll your eyes and leave a scathing review on Amazon, consider how you will react the first time you experience the pains of food poisoning... at midnight, during a thunderstorm, in the middle of a National Forest, with no toilet and three napkins. At that moment, you will be questioning all of the decisions that got you to this moment, and wondering what you could have done differently to avoid this very situation. It is from the perspective of that person, and for that person, that I wrote this book. Just a few years ago, that person was me, and I was hideously unprepared for the adventure to which I had committed myself.

Perfection is impossible, and disease is inevitable. However, by exercising calculated risk, and doing our best for ourselves, by ourselves, we can ride this van life adventure for as long as we wish. I wrote extensively about knowing how to be able to fix your van in my first book, **How to Live the Dream: Things Every Van Lifer Needs to Know.** The same concepts apply here, with your body and your mind.

I've kicked around what it means to be "successful" at van life, and at the end of the day, I think it boils down to this:

- Are you doing well? Mentally, physically, emotionally?
- Is the van still running?
- Do you have enough of what you need to survive?
- Are your emotional needs met?
- Do you wake up every morning feeling pretty good about your van life?

If you can answer yes to these questions on most days, then I'd say you're pretty successful. Congratulations, and here's to many happy travels in your van life!

# Resources

I like to include resources at the end of each of my books, because I love learning. I figure if you picked up a book with "How To…" in the title, chances are good that you love learning too. I don't actually know everything about everything, but I do a lot of research to write these books, which involves immeasurable time spent searching for reliable, current sources and effort reaching out to my van life buddies to learn about their experiences, as well.

This book, however, is unique. While some of the following links will lead to resources where you can get more information about a particular topic, others are educational sites that can enrich your knowledge about the topics covered in each chapter. If you want camp burner recipes, I've got links. If you want a great YouTube video to help your children learn about how your immune system works, I've included those types of links as well. Don't worry, everything is labeled, and I didn't include anything gory or questionable.

Having struggled with a chronic condition myself, I feel like knowledge gives us power over things that we can't necessarily control, but can mitigate and learn to live with.

I am in no way affiliated with any of these links, nor is anyone I know. I was not paid or reimbursed in any way for referencing them. These are simply resources I found in my own independent research, gathered, and included here because I felt they may be of use to other van folks and prospective van folks. I have no control or input into what is published in these links, either.

**What You Need to Know**
These are all educational links, pulled from peer-reviewed, scientific sources. As I started to write this book, I realized that I have no credibility on medical topics. I pay attention, I read, and I do a ton of research.

These links may be only vaguely referenced in the text, but I wanted to "show my work" in spots, to demonstrate that I'm not just inventing this information. The following represent some of the sites I used extensively throughout the planning and writing of this book. If these articles aren't relevant to your situation, I encourage you to search these resources for more information.

Germs vs Surfaces:
- *How long do nosocomial pathogens persist on inanimate surfaces? A systematic review* https://www.ncbi.nlm.nih.gov/pmc/articles/PMC1564025/

Keeping clean:
- *Cleaning and Disinfection* https://www.cdc.gov/mrsa/community/environment/index.html

How Antibodies Work:
- *Antibodies* https://www.newscientist.com/term/antibodies/

An Interesting Article about Epidemiology:
- *How Europeans brought sickness to the New World* https://www.sciencemag.org/news/2015/06/how-europeans-brought-sickness-new-world

**Preventive Care**

Preventive care is a bit of a pet topic for me, so I was very excited to include a chapter that focused on the basics. I also know that everyone is different, and comes from a different background. You are welcome to disagree with my assessments regarding preventive care. I've included a few links here so you can gather the information needed to make your own informed decisions.

Medical Checkups:
- *www.Healthline.com "How Often Should You See Your Doctor for a CheckUp"*

https://www.healthline.com/health/how-often-should-you-get-routine-checkups-at-the-doctor#benefits

Oral health care:
- *Centers for Disease Control and Prevention "Oral Health Tips"* https://www.cdc.gov/oralhealth/basics/adult-oral-health/tips.html

Vaccinations and travel considerations:
- https://www.vaccines.gov/who_and_when/travel
- https://wwwnc.cdc.gov/travel
- https://www.cdc.gov/rabies/transmission/index.html#:~:text=Rabies%20virus%20is%20transmitted%20through,bite%20of%20a%20rabid%20animal.

Maintenance medications:
- https://www.cdc.gov/nchs/fastats/drug-use-therapeutic.htm

**Insurance Considerations**

My mantra through this entire section was "don't write an entire book about insurance." That's not why you're here. That being said, I know that healthcare costs in the United States are very, very high. I know that most people on the road aren't making a sweet six-figure paycheck each week, either. I wanted to provide substantial information on the topic, so you can make informed decisions about what makes the most sense for you, your family, and your overall financial situation.

Emergency Room vs. Urgent Care Details:
- https://www.debt.org/medical/emergency-room-urgent-care-costs/

Shopping for individual health care plans:
For this particular exercise, I didn't want to provide just one option or view, so here are a few different links that can provide guidance through searching for a healthcare plan outside of employer benefits.

- How much Does Health Insurance Cost Per Month? https://www.healthmarkets.com/content/health-insurance-cost-per-month
- Online Healthcare Finder https://finder.healthcare.gov/
- Private Health Care Plans Outside Open Enrollment https://www.healthcare.gov/private-plan-exceptions-outside-open-enrollment/
- How to Buy Individual Health Care https://www.bcbsm.com/index/health-insurance-help/faqs/topics/buying-insurance/how-to-purchase-individual-health-insurance.html
- Guide to Buying an Individual Health Care Plan https://www.insurance.com/health-insurance/health-insurance-basics/how-to-buy-an-individual-health-plan.html

**Food and Nutrition**

All of these links lead to recipes and meal ideas. I can't vouch for how delicious, easy, or practical all of them are, because I used resources that included many ideas. I have tried many of them, and I feel pretty confident that there's at least one tasty, new meal option for you in at least one of these links! All of these are written with camping/boondocking in mind, which makes them particularly useful for those living the van life.

- From "Van Life UK Survivors Guide": https://www.vanlifeuksurvivorsguide.co.uk/post/how-to-never-get-bored-cooking-with-a-single-gas-burner-or-camping-stove?fbclid=IwAR0KbqV-15nOJ4lo-gei17BNB_BCFIJKSHBT9RTYYMh4-BSDQEn61n06ypEk
- My favorite campfire pizza: https://www.freshoffthegrid.com/campfire-pizza-recipe/
- Fantastic Mac and Cheese https://www.foodnetwork.ca/canada-day/photos/one-pot-camping-recipes/#!campfire-mac-and-cheese
- From "Fresh Off The Grid"" https://www.freshoffthegrid.com/camping-recipe-index/?fwp_activity=car-camping
- Food Network's Camping Hacks: https://www.foodnetwork.ca/

fun-with-food/photos/easy-camping-food-hacks/

**Exercise**

Believe it or not, I've tried nearly all of these. I'm not going to tattle on myself as to which I didn't do, but I will confirm that at one point, I was doing burpees next to the van to determine what would make them any easier. Being that I'm not a huge fan of burpees, that's a pretty subjective topic, but rest assured that a significant amount of conscientious research went into this chapter.

If you're doing any of these for the first time, please pay attention to the directions and details to avoid injury. Never exercise against the advice of your medical team. Take it easy, and honor your body. Most of all, have fun moving!

- *Outdoor Yoga Guidance and Routines*
  https://www.yogajournal.com/practice/call-of-the-wild
  https://www.doyou.com/your-guide-to-outdoor-yoga/

- *Yoga for Travelers (from Yoga with Adriene):*
  https://www.youtube.com/watch?v=C0U7v4iCemM

Specific Yoga Poses:
- *Warrior Pose:* https://www.mondaycampaigns.org/de-stress-monday/add-warior-yoga-pose-wellness-routine
- *Extended Triangle Pose:*
  https://www.yogajournal.com/poses/extended-triangle-pose
- *Extended Side Angle Pose:*
  https://www.youtube.com/watch?v=0IfzG9jH6cM&app=desktop
  https://www.instagram.com/p/BeZ0DDellwv/?utm_source=ig_share_sheet&igshid=ff45nb45b1gi

HIIT and Body Weight Exercise Tips:
- https://www.fitnessblender.com/videos/insane-hiit-challenge-bodyweight-only-high-intensity-interval-training-workout

- https://www.shape.com/fitness/workouts/lose-fat-fast-hiit-bodyweight-workout
- https://www.nerdfitness.com/blog/how-to-stay-in-shape-while-traveling/

Specific Cardio Exercises:
- *High Knees:*
  https://classpass.com/movements/high-knees#:~:text=High%20Knees%20are%20a%20cardio,a%20wide%20variety%20of%20workouts.
- *Squat Jumps:*
  https://www.youtube.com/watch?v=CVaEhXotL7M
- *Goblet Squats:*
  https://www.youtube.com/watch?v=MxsFDhcyFyE
- *Step-Ups:*
  https://www.youtube.com/watch?v=BeN9ZcYY5iM

Exercise and Wellness for Climbers and Hikers:
https://mountainmadness.com/resources/climbing-rating-systems
https://thetrek.co/8-best-stretches-thru-hikers/
https://jennybruso.com/unlikelyhikers/

**Managing Chronic Conditions**

I want to be as delicate and kind regarding various chronic conditions. All of them require a different level of maintenance, and each individual who lives with a chronic condition has their own experience. In my attempts to avoid making sweeping generalizations, I found that many resources do just that. From my own personal experiences, I am aware that living with Alzheimer's has different considerations than coping with cancer treatment, so I was pretty shocked to find that many sites just group every condition together.

The links that I've provided here provide some information about what chronic conditions are, and a few tips for managing them on the road. These tips seem to imply that people do not leave their home except in the face of disaster. The tips are solid for anyone who wishes to explore the world around them voluntarily, however.

A Definition of Chronic Conditions:
https://www.cms.gov/Research-Statistics-Data-and-Systems/Statistics-Trends-and-Reports/Chronic-Conditions/CC_Main

*How to Manage Your Chronic Disease During a Disaster*
https://www.cdc.gov/chronicdisease/about/manage/disaster.htm

*Chronic Disease in Uncertain Times*
https://newsinhealth.nih.gov/2020/08/chronic-disease-uncertain-times

## Dealing with Emergencies

This is another information-rich topic that I could wax on about all day, especially given my penchant for falling. The following links will help you prepare for the possibility of an emergency, and lead to further resources that can provide more extensive training and details than I could possibly fit in this book!

- *When to go to the ER:*
  https://www.healthline.com/health/right-care-right-time/where-to-go#1
- *What to do in an emergency:*
  https://www.webmd.com/heart-disease/features/5-emergencies-do-you-know-what-to-do
- *A thorough, printable first aid guide from Simple Family Preparedness:*
  https://simplefamilypreparedness.com/first-aid-quick-guide/
- *REI's Expert Guide to first aid kits (this section of REI's site provides a significant amount of information for van dwellers!):*
  https://www.rei.com/learn/expert-advice/first-aid-checklist.html
- *Things to keep in mind in case YOU are involved in an emergency:*
  https://www.health.harvard.edu/staying-healthy/are-you-prepared-for-a-medical-emergency

## Insect Management

You have a lot of options when it comes to taking care of the involuntary passengers you bring along on the trip. I consider this site a good introduction to the dilemma without forcing any potential ethical considerations. I know there are some humane and inhumane options when it comes to getting rid of pests, so I encourage you to work within your moral guidelines to keep infestations from happening.

https://www.boondockersbible.com/knowledgebase/how-to-keep-bugs-from-getting-into-your-rv/

## Laundry Day

Here are a few sites and a video that can address the question of how to do your laundry on the road. From choosing bio-friendly products to the actual steps involved, this should help you keep your clothes clean and in good repair while you're on the road. (Or hit a laundromat, if this isn't your forte!)

https://thecampingnerd.com/laundry-boondocking/
https://greatist.com/health/27-chemical-free-products-diy-spring-cleaning
https://www.youtube.com/watch?v=gePt65DyW2g

## The Immune System

With absolutely no disrespect intended, it has come to my attention that one can receive a significant amount of top-notch education and not know how the immune system works. There have been several times in my discussions with others that I have said, "but that's not how the immune system works," only to have to explain it. Not being a medical professional myself, I had to call in the experts for assistance. Hopefully, these links will help you as much as they have helped me.

https://www.ncbi.nlm.nih.gov/books/NBK279364
https://www.hopkinsmedicine.org/health/conditions-and-diseases/the-immune-system
https://www.youtube.com/watch?v=oqGuJhOeMek

## Online Therapy

Mental health is so incredibly important. As I was writing this book, nearly everyone I reached out to asked me to make sure I included a section about mental health. It's something that is frequently overlooked, especially when you're supposed to be having the time of your life. Living on the road has its own unique challenges, and while the van life community is incredibly supportive, sometimes it's best to call in a professional! Here are a few links to online therapy resources, as referenced in the text.

- *Talk Space:* https://www.talkspace.com/online-therapy/
- *Better Help:* https://www.betterhelp.com/start/
- *A Comprehensive List of Options:* https://www.verywellmind.com/best-online-therapy-4691206

These are not links exclusively for those living in a van. Absolutely anyone can use these links, as well as the emergency mental health contacts I've included within the text. Being a modern human being is complicated, so please don't feel ashamed to take advantage of any resource that can help you make it through rough times.

## COVID-19

We are absolutely bombarded with information about the COVID-19 pandemic of 2020, and hopefully, in the future, all of these links will be useless. For now, these are some frequently-updated sites that are helpful for travelers trying to make sense of van life rules and restrictions in an ever-changing landscape:

Tips for Travelers:
https://www.cdc.gov/coronavirus/2019-ncov/travelers/communication-resources.html
https://www.ustravel.org/toolkit/covid-19-resources-destinations
https://www.cnn.com/travel/article/us-state-travel-restrictions-covid-19/index.html

# Reviews

Reviews and feedback help improve this book and the author. If you enjoy this book, we would greatly appreciate it if you could take a few moments to share your opinion and post a review on Amazon.

## Also by Kristine Hudson

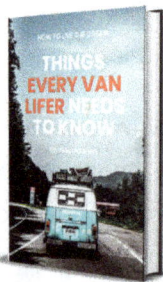

**Things Every Lifer Needs to Know**

mybook.to/vanlife

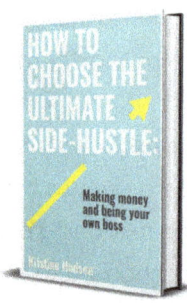

**How to Choose the Ultimate Side-hustle**

mybook.to/side-hustle

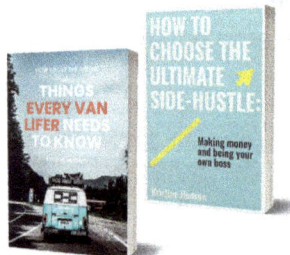

**The Modern Woman's Guide to Living Wild and Free**

mybook.to/vanbundle1

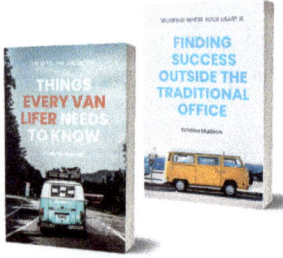

**Living and Prospering Wherever You Wish**

mybook.to/vanbundle2

www.ingramcontent.com/pod-product-compliance
Lightning Source LLC
Chambersburg PA
CBHW051544020426
42333CB00016B/2098